COMPASSION HEALS

COMPASSION HEALS

From Self-Care to Healthcare

August 16, 2021

LEE TOMLINSON

My dear dear Maria.
Wow. We've been thru
the grinder, right? But,
they can't keep us down!
We'll find ways to bring
more love and compassion

Waterside Productions

no matter what... Right?
with love + gratitude
"Patient" Lee Tomlinson

Printed in the United States of America

First Printing, 2021

ISBN-13: 978-1-951805-15-9 print edition
ISBN-13: 978-1-951805-16-6 ebook edition

Waterside Productions
2055 Oxford Ave
Cardiff, CA 92007
www.waterside.com

"Be kind, for everyone you meet is fighting a hard battle."

—Ian MacLaren

TABLE OF CONTENTS

PREFACE

People say it only takes one person to make a difference. That's proved all too true for me, as without the kindness and compassion of one incredible doctor and friend, I would not be alive today.

Not too long ago, I was battling Stage III+ throat cancer. I'd lost my business to two criminal partners, was losing my marriage, sold our beautiful home and fancy cars in an effort to combat the soaring debt that was rapidly drowning me, and had received indescribably cruel and dehumanizing medical treatment, leaving me feeling worthless, and more relevantly, hopeless. I had moved past contemplation and had formed a plan as to how I would end my life—an act I believed would bring an end not only to my suffering, but to the suffering I believed I had foisted upon those around me.

I am alive today because of a single compassionate act. Because of that gift, my life's mission is to inspire others, particularly in healthcare, to make compassion the anchor of both their professional and personal lives—to benefit their families, their colleagues, their companies; and perhaps most important, to benefit themselves.

My excruciating battle with near-fatal throat cancer made me painfully aware of the trauma caused by medical treatment lacking in compassion—indeed, it was the final straw that led me to consider taking my own life. What saved me from the darkest of depths was a tiny, simple, yet powerful act of compassion delivered by a loving friend.

This single act of compassion not only revived my will to fight and live, but also sparked within me an impassioned desire to devote myself to reconnecting as many people as possible with the immense and scientifically proven power of compassion to heal the minds, bodies, and souls of others, as well as themselves.

In these troubled times when anger, violence, and mayhem seem to be the norm, there is reason to wonder if all this compassion stuff really matters. I get it. If you're like me, it's really easy to slip into that cynical place where we lose faith in the belief that we can really make a difference anywhere, anytime. You might wonder if one person even has the ability to change or even save a life. You might doubt that that one person could be you.

What I do know is this: every moment you are in the presence of another human being, they are, at some level, in some kind of pain, which means that you always have an opportunity to make an impact, for better or for worse. To connect and uplift—or not. It's your choice.

CHAPTER 1

"Cure sometimes. Treat often. Comfort
always."

—Hippocrates

I'm Lee Tomlinson, a Stage III+ throat cancer survivor, and I'm very pleased and lucky to be alive
today.

I used to want to work in healthcare. I loved the
idea of it, loved the thought of being able to do my
part to help others and take away their pain. The
problem is that I've never had the stomach (or, if
we're being honest here, the brains) to do it. When
that sad fact presented itself, I turned my focus to
pursuing other goals, and that's worked out pretty
well for me. I've been a movie studio executive and
owner. I raised tens of millions of dollars for a major
charity as an award-winning television producer.
I've been a professional athlete and a TEDx Talk
presenter.

But now, because history has a funny way of
repeating itself, I find myself again fascinated by

and in awe of modern healthcare. So enamored, in fact, that I happily spend most of my time traveling the world to speak and interact with as many healthcare professionals as I possibly can. Why?

My mission in life today is to inspire healthcare professionals (HCPs) to return increasingly absent compassionate patient care to its rightful place at the forefront of modern healthcare. It is because of a single, small-but-mighty act of compassion delivered by a loving doctor and friend that I am alive today, and as a result, it's my intention to spend the rest of my time on this earth inspiring healthcare professionals to provide that same level of loving kindness to themselves so that they can better provide it to each and every one of their patients.

So what gives me the authority, the experience, the *right*, to talk to HCPs, when I could never hack it in the medical field? Simple. I'm a perpetual, lifelong patient.

It all started when I was five years old and my older sister dragged me up to the second story landing of the stairwell, pointed down the stairs, and yelled, "Prove it!" She was, of course, referring to my persistent declaration that I was not Mom and Dad's little boy, but rather the son of Superman. "Prove that you're the son of Superman or shut up about it," my sister said. And I did.

My parent's first thought was that she might have pushed me—not an unreasonable conclusion—but the truth is, I dove happily and without hesitation.

Just. Like. Superman. You might say I fell. I say I flew. I remember watching my parents' beautiful artwork mounted in the stairwell whiz past my face. I remember the feeling of flying. It was exhilarating.

Until I crashed.

I woke up the next morning encased in a white body cast with a severe concussion and a collarbone broken in three places. My mother sat beside me, weeping, with her hand on my arm to comfort me— something she did with painful-for-both-of-us regularity for the rest of her ninety-three-year life.

Since then, I've had a compound fracture of my left arm, broken more than a dozen bones— nose, shoulder, foot, and numerous fingers and toes—some as many as three times. I've had more infections and infectious diseases than I can count, including pneumonia and spinal meningitis; two near-fatal motorcycle accidents; I was rescued off the top of a mountain, as well as from drowning after being dared and doing a one-and-a-half flip off the side of a boat in the Dead Sea and being knocked unconscious when I hit my head on the bow. I've had hypothermia and heat stroke in the same year, had my thumb pulled off, my toe amputated, numerous skin grafts and bone grafts. Don't forget the four dog bites, horse bites and kicks...I could go on, but that wouldn't make for a very interesting book (unless you're into blood and guts).

The point is, I didn't remotely know what the heck the word compassion meant when I was young, but I sure as heck knew what it felt like when I was in pain and scared to death. It had nothing to do with my medical treatment, but it had everything to do with caring. Not what those HCPs *did* to me … but rather *how* they did what they did to me.

In all those years of being treated for a myriad of never-ending illnesses and injuries, I never gave compassion a thought. It wasn't until the darkest moments of my life, when I found myself without it, that I realized: all any of us wants when we're in pain is a little love and respect. And it wasn't until I finally received the compassion I so desperately craved in that darkest of times that I found myself with a deeper will to be a more compassionate person myself, and to share that will with the far too frequently burned-out healthcare workers who need it the most.

That was the moment I found my true mission, my reason for living. Why I was born. And my mission is very much like most of those same HCPs: to do whatever I can to relieve the suffering of those in pain, only my "patients" aren't those people admitted to healthcare centers across the globe—they're you. Now, my greatest goal in life is to inspire healthcare professionals to be more compassionate to themselves, to do what it takes to be healthy inside and out, so that they can give that same compassionate gift to their patients.

Life has come full circle for me. Rather than have the privilege of helping heal patients, I get to try to help healthcare professionals avoid the epidemic of HCP burnout, heal themselves, and *then* better heal others. In doing so, a dream comes true for me. I get to do what I've never gotten to do— help heal and care for each and every one of you out of my appreciation and thanks for treating *and* caring for me.

Given the proven fact that kindness and compassion are contagious[1]—that is, when given the gift of kindness, recipients tend to "pay it forward" and deliver another kind act to someone else in their life, then someone else, then someone else—it is, by its very nature, the gift that keeps on giving.

(By the way, every statement we make about the specific healing qualities, the value and impact of compassionate interactions has been proven through rigorous, peer-reviewed scientific studies. Don't worry, we will cite our sources.)

Will compassion transform the life of every person in the world? Maybe, maybe not. But we have to try, and never, ever give in to the cynical, negative voice that tells us that making a difference is impossible. Why? Because you can! It is absolutely possible.

Where there is life, there is breath. And where there is breath, there is hope. Hope for an even

---

1 "KINDNESS IS CONTAGIOUS, NEW STUDY FINDS." Shannon Mehner, Apr 21, 2010. https://helix. northwestern.edu/article/kindness-contagious-new-study-finds

better tomorrow than today. Let's make it so by being compassionate to everyone—starting with ourselves.

We have to start somewhere. Let's have it be today. Let's get people who are already committed to doing good, to do just a little bit more. For the ones on the fence, let's inspire them to move upward. And to our haters—they're probably just gonna stay haters. Too bad. But you know what? I'll wager that over time, we'll even get a few of them! Wanna bet?

CHAPTER 2

"I've learned that people will forget what
you said, people will forget what you did, but
people will never forget how you made them
feel."

—Maya Angelou

I have a confession to make. I have an addiction.
Not to drugs or alcohol. I'm addicted to adrenaline, and it's largely because of this addiction that
I've been in and out of medical care for so much
of my life. (Well, that plus some considerable bad
luck and not-so-great decisions.) It's because of that
adrenaline addiction that I've received the majority of my aforementioned injuries, experienced so
many adventures, and, most recently, jumped out of
a plane in celebration of my cancer remission (five
years, No Evidence of Disease [NED]. I'm statistically cured!). Blessedly, that adventure did not end
in hospitalization. More about that later. It's also this
addiction that led me into the capable hands of the
esteemed Dr. Franklin Ashley.

LEE TOMLINSON

When I was ten, my best friend and next-door neighbor invited me to go water skiing with him and his dad. I had only ever seen water skiing in photos and on TV, so naturally I was thrilled to go. My parents gave the OK, so one Sunday morning, we packed up our gear and headed up to Lake Piru in northern Ventura County, California.

Always eager for a thrill, I was impatient for my turn. If flying off the stairway taught me anything, air, intensity, and movement are things I love. Water skiing held a lot of attraction for me—like maybe I could recapture that feeling of flying. And, indeed, it seemed a lot like flying down the stairwell when I proved I *was* Superman's son—only this time on water.

I strapped on the skis as soon as I could, my neighbors started up their speedboat, and on my very first run, I made it up onto my skis—a major accomplishment. I was skiing! It was exhilarating! But then I hit a huge wave, and my hand got caught in the towrope. I pulled my arm back in an attempt to free myself, but the sudden motion caused me to lose my balance and slam into the water. The friction from the water stopped me almost immediately.

Unfortunately, the speedboat didn't receive the memo, and continued flying away at twenty-five miles per hour. The rope tightened instantly, and by the time I'd resurfaced, it had pulled off my thumb and much of the skin on my left hand.

The ensuing chaos is a bit of a blur, but I do remember the panic of my neighbor as they put on a tourniquet to stop the gushing bleeding, threw me in the back of someone's station wagon (a precursor to RVs for you youngsters), and frantically raced to find a doctor available on a Sunday afternoon in the middle of nowhere.

Our first stop was at the office of a local doctor whom I can only describe, all these years later, as an asshole. (Sorry for the obscenity, but true is true.) Insensitive, unkind, and totally uncaring, he grinned as he looked at my mutilated, thumbless hand and tear-streaked face and said, right in front of me, "Don't worry, it'll be fine. We'll just cut the rest of it off." He thought it was a joke. I thought my friend's dad was going to punch him in the face. If he had, I'd still be thumbless to this day. Thankfully, he didn't, and we sped off.

Eventually we ended up at Ventura County Hospital, where fortuitously there was an educational seminar being held for the resident doctors about a new surgical specialty called "reconstructive surgery." The man leading the seminar was none other than the legendary Dr. Franklin Ashley, who was in the process of creating the reconstructive surgery department at UCLA Health—one of the first in the world of its kind.

Somehow, the news of my plight made it to Dr. Ashley, who instantly decided that he would take me on as a new patient. Ventura County wasn't even his hospital; he just happened to be there at the moment I arrived, and the rest, as they say, is history. Thank God, he started my very first skin graft that day. All by pure chance. Just so I wouldn't go through life without an opposable thumb—a major disadvantage to a sports and adventure junkie like me. Despite having had my thumb pulled off, sometimes I think I have the best luck on the face of the planet. Actually, I know it.

As his practice grew, Ashley became widely known as the plastic surgeon to the stars, and he was a major hero of mine (not least because his list of famous patients included the legendary John Wayne, the hilarious barrier-busting female comedian Phyllis Diller, and the crazy talented and beautiful Ann-Margret—yowza). It was Ashley who, through a multiyear series of nearly a dozen surgeries involving multiple skin and bone grafts, rebuilt my thumb, a then unheard-of procedure for which I was an unknowing guinea pig. His work on my thumb was so revolutionary that it was all recorded on 16 mm film. Videos of my surgeries were used for decades to teach incoming surgeons at UCLA Medical Center and around the world how to reconstruct all sorts of body parts.

I was blessed for the first many years of my life to believe that medical treatment and compassionate care were one and the same. It was just the norm for me. My early experiences with healthcare always left me feeling medically cared for and cared about as a living, breathing human being, not just some dumb little kid with no thumb. It was due to these years of compassionate care that I felt loved, rather than shamed, when I found myself at the wrath of Ashley, years after my groundbreaking surgery. Forever seeking a thrill, I made the dumb decision to play a violent game of dodgeball, which, when I was slammed with the ball from close range, destroyed the thumb he'd broken barriers out of the goodness of his heart to create for me.

He. Was. Furious. Not because I'd destroyed his masterpiece, but because of the pain he knew it had caused me to reinjure myself, and because of the pain he knew it would cause me to repeat much of the reconstructive processes again. In short, he was livid because he cared—deeply. About *me*.

He did rebuild my thumb, and I approached the healing process with much more delicacy this time. My parents raised me by the Golden Rule: treat others as you want to be treated. That, I learned the hard way, includes, among other things, respecting the time and effort others put into treating and healing you. The hardest part? That doesn't just include people who were kind to me, but the mean, short-tempered, angry "jerks" I encountered as well. Everyone! Yikes. Tough to do, right?

It's probably no wonder that I became a compassionate care advocate, because the Golden Rule pretty much defines it. But I never connected health-care with anything so esoteric as "compassion." I had no idea they were even remotely related—probably, in no small part, because I had no idea what the word "compassion" even meant.

The truth is, my research and experience have revealed that pretty much everyone in healthcare *wants* to provide compassionate, patient-centered care. It's why they tell me the majority of them got into that crazy hard profession in the first place! The question is: What is compassion? The process of beginning to show compassion for oneself, then for patients, begins by learning to understand the answers to these questions.

When I deliver my keynote presentations, I ask my healthcare audiences this very question—and I've asked it now hundreds of times—they mostly hem and haw and then come up with the definition of empathy, which is to be aware of and feel the pain others are experiencing. And, for a patient, it feels good knowing that someone really "gets" our pain, especially our medical professionals because it makes us feel less alone.

But, as the Dalai Lama once said, "Compassion is empathy, combined with action." It requires a person to do something to help relieve the pain and suffering of another to transform empathy into compassion. The *Oxford English Dictionary* precisely defines "compassion" as "concern for the sufferings or misfortunes of others." *Merriam-Webster* adds, "...with a desire to alleviate it." With these working definitions in mind, I like to break down "compassion" a bit more into an understanding of two concepts: "suffering" and "comfort."

If you work in healthcare, you're in the suffering business. If no one is suffering, you're out of a job. So what is it? Is it just the lacerations, the cuts, the bruises, the broken bones? I suspect you, like our good friend Webster, know better. According to Webster, suffering is the experience of mental, emotional, physical, and often spiritual pain. How can you be in a hospital—as a patient or a provider—and not have emotional pain? It's the anguish, the loss, the grief. But you didn't get into healthcare to watch people suffer. You're in the business of healing—and comforting—to lessen or relieve their suffering.

Hippocrates, widely considered to be the father of modern medicine, spoke a lot about healers. Mind you, he didn't differentiate between oncology nurses, doctors, food service providers, administrators, valet parkers—if you are involved in any manner, shape, or form with the healing of a person in pain, you are a healer. Period.

Hippocrates said that healers have only three jobs, two of which are only part-time: "Cure sometimes. Treat often. Comfort *always*." Not just when they're nice to you, or when you're in a good mood or well-rested. No. Always. No matter what. It is not optional. If you're a healer, it is an absolute imperative. So, what is comfort?

The Latin *confortare*, from which the word "comfort" is derived, means "to strengthen greatly."

Webster says that "comfort" means to provide emotional support, strength, and hope, consolation in times of loss, and encouragement in challenging circumstances. It has nothing to do with *what* you do to patients and everything to do with *how* you do what you do to them. It's about how you make us *feel* while you're doing what you're doing to us.

In healthcare, there is an ever-increasing tendency these days to place the majority of the emphasis on treating and trying to cure physical ailments and injuries. Not on compassionate care.

Did you know that 50 percent of patients believe that healthcare professionals are not compassionate—not at all?[2] Zero! That means that 50 percent of patients are not receiving the compassion they deserve and need for the best, quickest outcomes. And *that* might just be the most hurtful reality in healthcare today.

Imagine the impact it would have, the kind of results we'd see, if we always remembered that taking care of people's mental and emotional needs is considered to be "integral" to ensuring maximally effective cancer treatment, as noted by the World Health Organization. And, it's reasonable to conclude that if it's "integral" for cancer patients' treatment, it

---

2   "Can 40 Seconds of Compassion Make a Difference in Health Care?" Dr. Stephen Trzeciak. 6 August 2018. https://knowledge.wharton.upenn.edu/article/the-compassion-crisis-one-doctors-crusade-for-caring.

must also be integral for every patient, regardless of their injury or illness. Considering and responding compassionately to a patient's psychosocial needs every time you walk into their room—*that's* comfort. And, according to the "father of modern medicine," it is every healer and every healthcare professional's full-time job!

Oh, I almost forgot to mention—one day, out of the blue, I met a baggage handler at a New Jersey airport with a thumb just like mine. What are the chances? He was half my age. He told me he'd had his cut off by an electric saw. What Ashley had done with me had paved the way. I helped him get a new thumb! How cool is that?

CHAPTER 3

"Never doubt that a small group of thoughtful, committed citizens can change the world. Indeed, it is the only thing that ever has."

—Margaret Mead

In 2019, Drs. Anthony Mazzarelli and Stephen Trzeciak of Cooper University Health Care released a revelatory book titled *Compassionomics: The Revolutionary Scientific Evidence that Caring Makes a Difference*, a thorough compilation of decades of studies seeking to prove whether treating patients with compassion does or does not make a discernible difference—not just in the physical well-being of their patients, but for the HCPs who treat them—and the bottom line of the institutions in which their lives interact.

The correlations they found between practiced compassion and improved patient outcomes were and still are utterly amazing to me. Among other benefits for patients, compassion reduces pain, expedites healing, lowers blood pressure, and helps alleviate depression and anxiety. One study included in their work concluded that patients' anxiety was measurably reduced when they received a message of empathy, kindness, and support that lasted just forty seconds. Forty seconds!

Hundreds of patient studies on the benefits of compassion in treating and healing patients have concluded that those who experience compassionate care also experience:

- A physical feeling close to pleasure
- A reduced desire for addictive painkillers
- An increase in hope and optimism
- An empowered immune system
- An increased will to live

I'll be honest, I've read and talked about these benefits a million times, but I'm still blown away. Every time I think about all of that miraculous stuff, I have to ask myself, *Why don't I give the gift of compassion every single chance I get? Why doesn't everyone? And why do nearly 50 percent of America's patients say they experience zero compassion from the HCPs who treat them? Zero!*

I'm embarrassed to admit it, but I think it's important to acknowledge, as I suspect my excuse will resonate with more than a few of you. You know what my answer is most often? "I forgot." "I was distracted." "Too busy." I was thinking about something else when the opportunity to be compassionate appeared. I was pissed, frustrated, depressed, burned-out.

Compassionomics cites a Pew Research Center study that found the following:

> Fully one-third of all Americans do not even consider compassion for others to be among their core values. These recent studies on the state of compassion in the general population are important new data points, but the backdrop for the data was established decades ago in a famous study conducted by renowned Princeton University psychologists John Darley and Daniel Batson. Their classic experiment— a study of compassionate helping—found signs of a compassion crisis way back in 1973, even among people from whom compassion is most expected.

One of my goals is to make providing compassion a priority, a natural habit, rather than something we think of as a chore, or worse, as a waste of time. Not only for healthcare professionals in the course of treating patients and dealing with colleagues, but for everyone.

Close your eyes for a minute. Well, finish reading this paragraph first, then do it. Take a deep breath. Relax. Remember when you were five or six. What did you do when you got a nasty booboo? Close your eyes. Picture it.

Are they open again? They must be, if you're reading. Well, what did you do? Did you run to the emergency room? Tell the nearest stranger you had a severe laceration and ask them to call 911? No. You ran to your mom, or dad, or other person you thought you could trust. Right?

Of course you did. We all did. And what did you want first? A hug and kiss to make it all better. Right?

That's comfort. Remember what *Merriam-Webster* taught us: it's the care and attention to the psychosocial needs of others—not the physical treatment—that brings us comfort. Let me give you another example.

Some years ago in September 2009, Army Captain William D. Swensen was involved in a mission in the Ganjgal Valley in Eastern Kunar Province, Afghanistan. His 160-man squadron of soldiers was pinned down by enemy fire, while surrounded on three sides by enemy troops. In the middle of that battle, a fellow soldier, Sergeant Kenneth Westbrook, was shot in the neck. Without even pausing to put on his helmet, Swenson grabbed his fallen colleague, slung him over his shoulder, and ran 150 yards in soft sand through intense enemy fire to bring the man to a helicopter for evacuation.

That's incredible in and of itself, but it wasn't enough for Swenson. He wanted to do more than just get his colleague's horrific wound treated—fast.

He wanted to comfort the man whose life he was trying to save as well. Once the injured man had been safely dropped into the helicopter, at great risk of losing his own life, Swenson had the presence of heart and mind to give Westbrook a loving hug and kiss on the forehead before running back into the warzone. It took a nanosecond, but I'm certain that the soldier and comrade he saved remembered that moment for the rest of his life. Swenson was later awarded a Medal of Honor for his simple but profoundly kind act. There's even an incredible video capturing it; I show the clip at all of my talks. If you'd like to see it, go online and do it.[3] I promise you will be deeply moved by this simple act of compassion.

And we all think we don't have time to be compassionate. "I'm too busy." This story alone proves that wrong—let alone all the clinical studies. With compassion, small is all. And even the smallest of loving gestures is enough to show you really care about someone.

That's comfort, too, and comfort is just another name for compassion. We may not all be able to relate to the feeling of being rescued in combat with a fatal injury, but we all know the sensations of warmth and security associated with being comforted; of getting that proverbial or literal hug and

---

3   https://youtu.be/en1ZHMANDkg

kiss from someone who cares about us when we're hurting. So, how do you know if you gave that feeling of comfort to others?

Over the years, I've done an enormous number of interviews, primarily of cancer patients and HCPs. I've asked my fellow patients to share their experiences with healthcare professionals, the details of their medical treatment, and when they felt the most and least comforted. From all the qualitative data I gathered, I've managed to identify four behaviors that, when combined, create an overall feeling of compassionate care.

Creative Health Care Management, or CHCM, is a heart-driven organization that has been paving the way for what they call "Relationship-Based Care," a.k.a. compassionate care, in the healthcare industry for decades. They are wonderful, intelligent, compassionate people, and I can't recommend them, or their books, seminars, and classes, highly enough.

As is often the case with people who have devoted their lives and careers to working in the healthcare industry—one of the many reasons I admire them so very much—is they've figured out how to concisely define the four components of comforting, compassionate care far better than I could ever have phrased it on my own. CHCM CEO and nurse Mary Koloroutis and psychologist Michael Trout coauthored the book *See Me as a Person* in which they define four *therapeutic* practices to connect with patients as unique persons and interact with compassion and care.[4] These practices do not take more time, they facilitate connection in the moment. In order to know you've provided the most compassionate care of which you're capable, Koloroutis and Trout recommend asking yourself if you provided the following four actions while attempting to provide comfort and relieve someone's pain:

The next time you want to know whether or not you have been compassionate when interacting with a patient, ask yourself the following questions:

· **Did I ATTUNE—connect with myself before connecting with the patient? Did I give the patient my full attention and focus on their current state?**
We cannot connect meaningfully with others unless we are tuned-in to ourselves. When we pause and take a breath, we make space for greater connection with others. Attuning is the practice of being present in the moment, not with the last person we were with, and not with the one after this one. Rather, it's about "tuning in" to ourselves and then others. When we attune to patients, we are meeting them exactly where they are and remembering that what might be routine for us is often life-altering

---

4   Koloroutis, Mary, and Michael David Trout. 2012. *See Me as a Person: Creating Therapeutic Relationships with Patients and Their Families.* Minneapolis, Minn.: Creative Health Care Management.

for them. Try this: Before entering a patient room, pause for a moment, take a mindful breath, let it out and as best you can, slow down. Then connect with the patient/family with a focus on their state of being (physical, emotional, mental, and spiritual).

Learning to attune fosters a greater connection with others. Did you first take a moment for yourself, then look your patient straight in the eye? Did you know their name? If you've seen this person before, did you remember them? Do you know anything about their personal history? Did you take the five seconds to ask them? If this was your first time meeting, did you introduce yourself?

· Did I WONDER what my patient could teach me about themselves? Was I open-minded? Do I remember that everyone has a unique backstory? Did you use your patient's preferred salutation: Mr., Ms., and so forth? Did you use their desired pronouns? Did you greet them and answer any questions they may have had before beginning a medical procedure? Did you say "please" and "thank you?" (Our parents called them "magic words" for a reason.) Did you show genuine interest in your patient's story and needs?

Unless we're careful, we often unconsciously make assumptions about others when we meet them which are, more often than not, inaccurate. And, if we interact with them according to those inaccurate assumptions, those with whom we interact will feel unseen and unheard and anything but comforted. Wondering is the practice of bringing an open-hearted curiosity toward others by recognizing and suspending assumptions and judgment. It is the practice of being genuinely interested in them and understanding that only patients can tell us about their wants, needs and fears. Their input is critical to quality care.

> Try this: Be curious about what your patient will teach you. Be curious about your patient's backstory and how it is impacting their interactions and responses to care. Ask them about their lives outside the hospital, their families, hobbies, history, careers. And, next time you see them, remember those stories and bring them up. That's what makes someone feel special, and genuinely seen, heard, and appreciated. You may not learn everything about them, but the point is to show you care by asking—and you may learn something that is very important to the provision of care.

· **Was I FOLLOWING the trajectory of my patient's needs? Did I follow my patient by staying present and truly listening?**
Did I listen to what mattered most to them? If it's cold in the room, offer your patient a blanket. Ask if they're thirsty and offer a drink of water. If there's a language barrier, consider enlisting a multilingual

colleague who may be able to assist. And if they just need some encouragement that everything's going to be all right, stay with them and provide that encouragement. I know you're crazy busy, without a lot of extra time. But remember that kiss on the forehead of his mortally wounded fellow soldier from Army Captain William D. Swenson? How long did that take? Two seconds! It's all about connection, not time.

Once we inquire and find out about people's personal wants and needs, the real gift is interacting with them in ways that reflect your knowledge of those specific needs. Do they want to be called by their first or last name? Do they have a preference as to whether or not you knock before you enter? Is the perfect room temperature higher or lower? Do they prefer coffee or tea? Do they like the shades open or closed? And, if we take note of these preferences and supply them, the recipient will absolutely feel comforted because you've clearly put their needs first, not yours. That is hugely calming and comforting.

> Try this: next time you are with a patient or family member, ask questions about them, listen to and validate their answers, then make sure they get as many of their preferences as humanly possible.

· **Did I "HOLD" them?**
Koloroutis and Trout explain this last point this way: "When we hold an infant, we instinctively cradle

them in our arms. Holding a patient is the same thing but from a psychological perspective."

Did you go through the motions like an automaton, or were you genuine and deliberate? Did you allow the patient the opportunity to express themselves? Did you express your own joy, curiosity, or interests? Did you attune, wonder, and follow?

"Holding a patient is the same thing but from a psychological perspective. It is the practice of intentionally creating a safe haven that protects the dignity of an individual. It is the practice of speaking with respect for them as persons."

> Try this: next time you are caring for an angry or distressed patient, experiment with remembering that anger is a normal human response to illness. It comes from feelings of fear and powerlessness. Acknowledge their feelings, remain a sturdy and compassionate presence, and take kind actions to ease their suffering.

If you've answered yes to all four of the questions above, then you've delivered what I call the CARE Effect.

I like to think of the CARE Effect as just another synonym for compassion. Just like any other skill, it takes a lot of practice and intention, but once you've gotten in the habit of asking yourself these four questions and you've committed to being compassionate, it becomes almost automatic. The best part? It becomes second nature to deliver the CARE Effect, a.k.a. compassion, to everyone—from patients to colleagues to relatives to strangers on the street.

CHCM believes that all healthcare professionals should be guided by a shared purpose to reduce suffering and bring more psychosocial connection to work in the healthcare industry. The four practices of attuning, wondering, following, and holding are critical skills that when incorporated into your daily practice, will show significant improvement in the quality of patient care and reduced signs of burnout in HCPs—and the ability to evaluate whether you have shown compassion to others will serve you well outside of healthcare, too.

One night, I was wandering back to my hotel from a rehearsal for a keynote address at a major medical conference, and I found myself lost. (This happens more often than I'd care to admit.) The hotel was only three blocks from the venue, so I knew I couldn't have gotten too far off track. I ambled up to two women who were walking ahead of me, intending to ask for directions. I said, "Excuse me," and was about to ask them for directions when I noticed that one of them looked very upset. Her body language was stiff, and her face was red and teary-eyed as if she'd been crying. "Can you tell me where the hotel is?" I asked, but as soon as she opened her mouth to answer, it was clear—she had definitely been crying. "Excuse me," I said, "But, are you okay?"

She looked at me as if to determine whether or not I posed a threat as well. "No," she finally told me. "Some guy just ran up and racially insulted me. He came out of nowhere, and it scared the hell out of me."

Well, what do you suppose we ended up doing? First, I asked her if he was still around and if they needed physical protection. They said they didn't think so. Then I asked if she wanted me to walk them where they were going just to be sure. They gratefully declined and then we just hugged for about thirty seconds there on the street. I'd never met this woman in my life, and she didn't know me from Adam, but I promise you that by the time I continued on my way, she was calmer, less upset, and…somewhat comforted because someone actually cared about her. And you know what? So was I. No kidding. I felt great, too. As upsetting as her experience was, at least I'd done something to try to make up for what she'd experienced and it was clear that we both felt better for it.

We all have deep pain: mental and emotional. We've all experienced some form of loss and grief. Everybody could always use a bit of comfort and compassion. Everybody craves it. And it takes just a nanosecond. Every moment is an opportunity, because every human being on this planet is fighting a great battle. We all have pain—we just need to be willing to look at it, feel it, and admit to it. When we are given the gifts of kindness, caring, and compassion when we really need it, we're likely to remember it for the rest of our lives. We will not remember all of the details of the radiation, the vaccination, or surgery, but we will remember a proverbial loving hug and kiss from someone who genuinely cares about us, I promise you. That's what heals us. The rest just cures us. And both, from a patient's perspective, are equally important. It's not enough to be merely technically competent with a patient—you have to be competent *and* compassionate to give your patients the best chance of healing and a cure.

That feeling of comfort is the first memory called to mind when I think of Dr. Michelle Putnam, my dear ENT (ear, nose, and throat specialist) and allergist. I have a million allergies—you name it, I'm allergic to it—but, when I sped into the parking lot outside her office on June 23, 2012, (10:28 a.m., but who's counting?) I was not happy. I love my doctors, nurses, and other HCPs—after all I'm alive because of them—but I hate going to see them. Why? Because more often than not, I'm going because I'm in pain, or they're going to do something that will hurt me, or ready me for something that's going to hurt me in the future. But this appointment was important because it had to do with my other addiction. No, not to adrenaline. Golf. Yup. I'm totally addicted. Embarrassing, but true.

So on this particular day, as usual, I was not looking forward to my visit, but this was an emergency. My allergies were far worse than ever, and that's saying something. I take a ton of medicines for them, but I was pretty sure a new one had appeared, and that was just not okay. You see, I had recently qualified for the California State Senior Amateur Golf Championships held in Monterey, California, home to Pebble Beach—the pinnacle of courses for golfers worldwide—and here I was unable to breathe, nose and ears painfully congested, eyes watering. I knew I wouldn't be able to play, let alone compete at a high level, if I couldn't see, hear, or breathe. And I darn well wasn't going to let some stinking new allergies get in the way of me and the state championships. Not a chance! So, I took an early lunch break and made a last-minute appointment with my trusted ENT for an allergy test. By the way, guess what I was allergic to? Grass. Yup. Seriously? Grass? A golf addict allergic to grass? That's just not fair! The universe has some twisted sense of humor. Not! (Later, my wife semi-laughingly said it was God's way of punishing me for spending so much time on the course instead of with her. Frankly, there's probably some truth in that.)

Anyway, once the initial exam was completed and Dr. Putnam had finished laughing about the irony of my newly discovered allergy, she asked me the question that would forever change the course of my life: "Lee, do you mind if I do one more test?"

Yes! Absolutely, I minded.

Dr. Putnam's office was located just down the street from the famed Culver Studios, which my partners and I had purchased from Sony Pictures Studios some years before. Built in 1918, Culver is one of the oldest continually operating studios in Hollywood history. It has been owned and operated by the likes of Cecil B. DeMille, Joseph P. Kennedy (father to Jack and Robert), Howard Hughes, Lucy and Desi Arnez, and a host of others. It's where iconic films like *Gone with the Wind*, the original *King Kong*, *Rocky*, *Citizen Kane*, *Raging Bull*, and *E.T.* were filmed and equally iconic TV shows like *The Andy Griffith Show*, *Lassie*, *Batman*, *Superman*, *Arrested Development*, *Mad About You*, and *Cougar Town* were shot. When we bought it, it was a mess, and we worked hard for years to bring it back to profitability.

From the outside, my life looked perfect. I was relatively well-to-do, successful, and married to the love of my life. In reality, my life was a brutal, stressful mess on all fronts.

A couple of years prior, I caught my partners embezzling a ton of money from the studio. When I confronted them one evening, they went ballistic. Between night and morning, security was told that if I was let onto the grounds, they'd lose their jobs, and I was locked off the lot. They stopped paying me and forged our partnership contract (with the help of their attorney!) to eliminate me (and another of our partners) from the partnership. I had no other option but to sue.

If you happen to know firsthand, my deepest sympathies; lawsuits are incredibly expensive. Crushingly so. I was using my own money to fight my case and was no longer receiving my generous six-figure salary. My former partners were using the studio's money. In discovery, they spent seven days interviewing me for ten hours a day about anything they could (yet nothing of consequence), knowing that ten hours a day at my lawyer's five-hundred-dollar-per-hour rate would kill me. They were right that it put me in the red, but they didn't count on my stubbornness. A week before the trial, knowing that they couldn't win, they settled with me. I ended up with their ownership interests in the studio, making me a significant equity owner of the famed Culver Studios. Pretty, pretty cool for a guy who truly *loved* great movies and had created, funded, and executive produced a decade of highly profitable three-hour Primetime CBS Specials for the American Film Institute that identified and celebrated the one hundred greatest movies and movie stars from the first century of American cinema. Many of which were shot at Culver!

Unfortunately, Lehman Brothers owned the rest of the property, and they wanted to own it in its entirety. No sooner had I won the suit against my former partners than Lehman reached out and demanded that I sell to them what I'd just won from my former partners. Okay, fine. I asked them to make me an offer, and they did, at a fraction of its value, which would have left me hundreds of thousands of dollars in the hole. I'd just spent two years battling the lawsuit. I turned them down.

That's when Lehman Brothers threatened to sue me as part of the partnership that defrauded them. "But I had nothing to do with this fraud. You know that! That's why I won my lawsuit." They didn't care.

So they sued me. I spent another two years fighting with Lehman Brothers on a case that had no merit, against an organization that had more money than God. They deposed me for a week as well. It all came to an end when they went bankrupt in the crash of 2008, one month before the trial they had zero chance of winning. Unfortunately, all of my ownership went into receivership, and I lost everything.

If you're at home keeping track, my wife and I were now deeply in debt. We sold our house to pay for the legal expenses (and to live, because I hadn't been drawing a salary now for nearly four years).

I still had a nice car, a decent place to live, and I was still hobnobbing with big movie stars. I had all the trappings of success, but the reality was I had no career, I'd wasted four years of my life in lawsuits, I ended up winning and losing everything in the same breath, and other than bankruptcy, I had no idea what to do. I was trying desperately to revive my career, my family, and my marriage required my full attention, and I was trying to focus on all of them at the same time—but there are only so many hours in a day. And frankly, I was beyond exhausted, deeply depressed, beaten up, and burned-out to a crisp.

So on that day in Dr. Putnam's office, I told her, with perhaps less than a gracious amount of patience, that I had to get back to work reinventing myself and working my way out of the mess I was in. "One more little test. It won't hurt, and it'll only take a few minutes," she said. Yeah, right. How many times had I heard that? It's never true. But I love her, trust her, and what the heck? A few minutes later, she had numbed me up for an "endoscopy."

Now, despite all my medical catastrophes, the only "-oscopy" I'd heard of was a colonoscopy, and I couldn't figure out why she wanted to give me one of those!

Turns out, an endoscopy is sort of like a colonoscopy, only starting at the other end. Dr. Putnam numbed my nose and throat with some spray and then inserted a wire with a camera on the end up my nose, then down my throat, and I tried to remain relaxed as I listened to her describe the procedure.

Let me make something crystal clear—when we patients put our lives in the hands of healthcare professionals (which in fact we do every time we see them, no matter the issue), we're always on high alert—fight or flight. Why? Deep down, we're terrified! It's not an issue of trusting, or not trusting, our healthcare providers so much as it's a primal fear that they'll need to do something that will hurt us or find something that could kill us. So we're paying very close attention both to what you're doing to us and how you're doing it. We see and feel everything acutely.

So as I sat there on high alert, watching Dr. Putnam perform the endoscopy on me, she suddenly took a sharp intake of breath, like something surprised her. I don't know about you, but I can only think of two sounds I never want to hear in a doctor's office. One is "oops," and the other is an abrupt, startled gasp.

"Lee, I don't know how to tell you this," Dr. Putnam said as she turned to me. I saw deep, deep sadness in her face. I tried to steel myself for whatever came next, but in hindsight there's no way I could ever have been prepared to hear her next words, "I think you have throat cancer."

"Wait, what?" What! I'm an athlete. A mountain climber, marathon runner, ex-professional athlete, and thrill seeker. I never drank, I never smoked. (Well, not tobacco. I did live in San Francisco in the '70s and '80s, after all, so maybe I did smoke a little you-know-what...but I swear I never inhaled. [If that story is good enough for a former two-time president, it's good enough for me and I'm sticking to it!]) The thought that I had cancer was inconceivable to me. I said, "That's impossible," but Dr. Putnam simply shook her head and with what looked like tears in her eyes said, "Lee, I am 99 percent sure that you do. I can see it right here," she said, pointing to the photo she'd taken of the tumor. "I would bet my career on it."

That's when I decided I was dead. My life was over. Done. My father had died of cancer. Both my grandmother and grandfather had died of cancer. Everyone I knew who had been diagnosed with cancer was dead. I had none of the risk factors to indicate I was at a higher degree of possibility for throat cancer, and I got it anyway. The reason? "Bad luck," according to my oncologists. No kidding.

I was stunned. I couldn't speak. Dr. Putnam was patient, waiting until I summoned the courage to ask my most important question: "Am I gonna die?" She reached out, put her hand on my arm, and softly, with a kind smile on her face said, "Yes... but hopefully not from this."

Needless to say, I didn't make it to the state championships. Later, when I met my oncologists, I asked if I could delay treatment in order to play. "No!" They responded in forceful unison. This was truly life threatening, and every day I delayed treatment, my chances of remission or a cure shrank. Hardheaded, macho guy that I was, I just didn't get it. This cancer was, literally, deadly serious.

I have to tell you, at that point in my life it was the worst news I'd ever gotten by a thousand miles. But what I remember most vividly—even more so than my abject terror—was that Dr. Putnam canceled several hours of responsibilities, told me to call my wife and get her over to her office, and then spent the next two hours patiently and lovingly addressing every question and concern we had.

Finally, as we got up to leave, Dr. Putnam handed me her business card. I remember thinking that was weird, since she'd been my ENT for fifteen years. Why would I need that? Until I looked at the card.

She'd crossed out the office phone number and written her personal cell phone number in its place. "You guys call any time of the day or night. For anything," she said. "The three of us are a team. I've got your backs. We're in this together!"

And yup, she gave each of us a warm hug and a kiss on the cheek.

She also told me that the next year of treatment would be the "hardest year of my life"—a strong contender for the understatement of the century—but I left her office feeling a little bit hopeful. Where three hours before I had been convinced that I was going to die, I now thought, maybe not. Why? Only because she attuned to *me*, she wondered about *my* health and *my* needs, she followed up with *me*, and through it all, she held and supported *me*. In short, because she cared. About me! Had she treated me? No. Had she cured me? No. Had she comforted me? Absolutely.

CHAPTER 4

"Compassion makes the unbearable, bearable."

—Dr. Kenneth Schwartz

As bad as I thought my cancer treatment was going to be, it was ten times worse. My life literally stopped. I could not muster the strength to even get out of bed. I stopped eating. I could not imagine working again. I could not imagine living through the experience.

Over that next year, Dr. Putnam continued to be a great source of support for me, as were brothers Eli and Ari Gabayan—the brilliant fraternal oncologists who oversaw my radiation and chemotherapy treatment. It was these two extraordinary men, founders of the famed Beverly Hills Cancer Center, that Dr. Putnam unreservedly recommended to me as my wife and I left her office that fateful day. Lucky me.

When I first met the Gabayans, there were three treatment options they proposed: surgery, then chemo, then radiation, in that order. The problem was that given the position of my tumor at the base of my tongue, there was a strong likelihood that surgery meant I would lose some or all of my tongue, and so lose my ability to speak. At the time, I was still a TV producer and in the entertainment industry; totally motivated by the art of the deal. And being that it's very difficult to strike a deal without a voice, I refused to even consider the recommended surgery. I already feared that cancer would take my life; I wasn't prepared to allow it to take away my ability to make a living, too—on the off-chance I survived.

"Surgery's not an option, guys," I said. "I can't lose my voice. I might as well already be dead. What's my next best option?"

I'll never forget the way they looked at each other, convinced that I still just didn't "get it," that I didn't understand how serious and potentially deadly this disease was. Finally, after a lengthy silence, they told me that the only alternative was to give me as much chemo and radiation as I could possibly bear. "And because you're so physically fit, if it doesn't kill you," they said not mincing words, "maybe we can avoid surgery."

I was really, really fit and healthy—cancer notwithstanding—and I guess they figured I could handle it. Thus began three months of chemo, followed by thirty-five straight days of radiation. Throughout the entire process, the Gabayan brothers and their staff were deeply compassionate and supportive, but

I would be remiss not to acknowledge my incredible oncology nurses and radiologic technologist as well.

I'll never forget my last month of chemo, when I found myself incapacitated on a weekend by the most persistent and continuous nausea I'd ever felt. Not at all uncommon with chemotherapy. The anti-nausea medicine they'd provided me for just such an occasion may as well have gone in the trash for all the good it did me. I had never felt more nauseated. I called the Gabayans' office, but their answering service was out of order and no one would pick up.

When I showed up on Monday morning for my next infusion, I was exhausted and miserable from non-stop vomiting. It's no small wonder that I didn't upchuck on the drive over.

Sure enough, though, as soon as they hooked up my drip, I started to vomit again. I had just enough time to grab a trash bucket and stick my head in it, but I threw up so violently and for so long that I swear I coughed up stuff I ate in the sixth grade.

It was horrible. Suddenly, in the depth of my misery, I felt myself surrounded by what felt like a host of angels. Instantly, I found myself in the loving embrace of four infusion nurses, led by the wonderful Lexi Timmons, who threw their arms around me in a warm hug, all the while whispering in my ear that I would be okay, that they were there for me, and that they weren't going to leave until I felt better.

After what seemed like forever, the retching finally subsided and I was able to look them in their loving eyes and silently thank them for their fierce comfort. Not surprisingly, that was an experience I will never, ever, ever forget. *That* is compassion. *That* is comfort.

Thank god for them, because never in all my years as a patient had I experienced anything like the misery and pain, on all levels, of cancer treatment. Cancer was every injury of my lifetime together, times a thousand. It made me weep. It kicked me, knocked me down, spit on me. Cancer insulted me, humiliated me, filled my neck, tongue, and mouth with sores. Nausea, excruciating pain, dizziness, sweating, freezing chills, migraine headaches—any possible side effect, I had it in the extreme. Towards the end, I couldn't eat, drink, or speak. I couldn't swallow. Swallowing simple saliva was like swallowing broken glass, so deeply damaged was my esophagus from thirty-five straight atomic blasts to my tender mouth and throat. I had hallucinations. By the time I was nearing the end of my thirty-five radiation treatments, I was literally living in fifteen-minute increments. Could I hang on from 1:15 to 1:30? From 1:30 until 2:00? Obviously, I did; I'm still alive. But toward the end, I wasn't sure I could or even wanted to. Kind, caring, compassionate people like my oncology nurses, radiology team, doctors, and everyone else at Beverly Hills Cancer Center got me through it. But what always happens when things seem like they can't get any worse? Yep. Things got worse. Way, way worse.

Toward the end of my treatment, I woke up in a hospital with what was for a while an unidentifiable and potentially fatal septic infection at the site of my port, surgically implanted in my chest. My loving wife was working hard trying to keep us solvent and couldn't always be there to keep me company. I hadn't worked in years, had acquired overwhelming quantities of debt due to my treatment and resultant lack of income, and was still unable to keep down most food and drink because of the excruciating pain brought on by simply swallowing. I was sick, lonely, and afraid. If ever there was a time in my life when I could have used the slightest bit of kindness, compassion, and comfort, it was then, in that "Hospital from Hell" where I was being treated. And I got zero. In fact, I got the exact opposite.

First off, the hospital was littered with dead plants, and let me tell you, the last thing anyone wants to see in a hospital is anything dead. If they can't keep an orchid alive and don't even notice the plants long after they obviously died, what could I expect from them? After being wheeled to my room, I discovered a long, black hair on the wall of my shower—obviously not mine, since I was bald as a cue ball from chemo—along with Jake, the strong and silent newt by the side of my bed who became my constant companion for three days, at which point I realized that he, like the plants, was dead.

Or so, despite our long, fentanyl-induced talks, the housekeeping staff told me.

As if the unsanitary conditions of my room weren't bad enough, the people were even worse: there was my phlebotomist, who never introduced herself; just came in, jammed in the needle, drew my blood, and exited wordlessly. There was the nurse who continually entered my room without knocking, even though I asked ten days in a row to please knock first, because due to my infection-induced 103.6°F fever, I was so hot some days I took my gown off to try to cool down. Worse, when I pleaded with her to do so, she said most patients didn't mind— implying I was being unreasonable!

There was the doctor who, while readying himself for the procedure of taking out my port, brutally bawled out the nurse assisting him, which deeply embarrassed her and scared me because he was so insensitive and unkind to her! The doctor was in such a great rush that he started cutting the port out before the numbing shots had taken effect. I screamed in agony. I yelled at him to stop, told him the pain was excruciating, begged him for more anesthesia. His response? "Hang on, I'll have it out in a second"—and he kept right on cutting it out then suturing the wound. It wasn't a second; it felt like hours, and when he finished, I was in terrible pain, exhausted, and drenched in sweat.

When I say that the employees of this hospital were the cruelest healthcare professionals I've ever encountered, I do not use that word lightly. I say it with no trace of exaggeration or drama. The medical professionals tasked with bringing me back from the brink of death were the most robotic, insensitive, impolite, and uncaring people I've ever met; totally lacking in compassion and simple human kindness.

And here's the thing. When we patients put ourselves into your hands, you control whether we live or die. You become gods to us. And when a god decides we're not worth so much as basic human kindness, we assume the problem is with us. We're not deserving. We're not good enough. We're not worth it. We did something wrong. We're a burden, a problem. I certainly believed as much. It was at this point that I began to have serious doubts as to whether I even wanted to continue the fight to live.

Luckily, they did manage to effectively treat my infection, and on the day that I was to be released, they sent me a "thank-you note" for choosing their hospital, at which I'd spent nearly one hundred thousand dollars. It arrived in a used envelope upon which they'd whited out the name of the previous recipient. Guess I wasn't worth the cost of a new envelope. They also managed to spell my name wrong: "Tomlison," not "Tomlinson." And the coup de gras: they'd addressed it to *Mrs.* Tomlison, not to Mr. They couldn't even get my sex right. Seriously? I felt totally miserable, unseen, and unheard. Totally alone.

My last round of chemo had concluded a few months prior, and I was in the last of my thirty-five straight days of radiation. Through a combination of an inability to work and uncovered medical expenses, we were running on empty. I was dying of cancer…and now the infection. I was in agony. The simple act of swallowing saliva was excruciating, and I literally stopped doing it for hours on end. I had lost nearly sixty pounds from my inability to eat or drink, and if I lost one more pound, my oncologists warned that they'd have to stop my treatment. The pain was so intense and so constant that I was given access to massive amounts of fentanyl patches—a hundred times more powerful than morphine and highly addictive—which barely dulled the pain. I was miserable. If these people, whose job it was to heal and treat the sickest and weakest of patients, didn't even care enough to simply be kind to someone in my condition, then what was the point of it all? I knew then, definitively, that I was a burden to them and everyone else in my life. To my loving wife, family, friends, colleagues, partners. All of them. Yup—a total burden. I was at such an emotional nadir I was no longer Lee Tomlinson, the fellow with a life and career and family. I was just some old guy in room 2212 with advanced cancer and a life-threatening infection. I was defined by the burden I had become. My continued existence was, itself, a cancer—or so I came to think after the inhumane treatment I had received.

It was then that I remembered the studio had taken out a Key Person Life Insurance policy on me worth a ridiculous amount of money—far more, frankly, then I could possibly imagine I was worth— pre-cancer or during. When I died, my wife would have enough money to erase all of our debt, and still live a life of luxury for the rest of her years—and not have to put up with me. My final parting gift. Perfect!

That was the final straw. I was about to be sent home and continue to self-administer my fentanyl patches. It occurred to me that if I put on enough of them, I would go to sleep, not wake up, and all our problems would be solved. Only one problem: I didn't know how many patches to use. If I put on too many, the coroner would rule my death a suicide, and my family couldn't collect on the insurance policy. Put on too few and I'd lapse into a coma and become an even bigger burden. I had to get this right and ask someone the right amount to get the job done and make it look like an accident.

Who better than a good friend who also happens to be a doctor, a former pioneering and immensely popular national talk radio and TV show host, and my brother-in-law, Dr. Dean Edell. If the name sounds familiar, it should—he was nicknamed "America's Doctor" before Dr. Oz took over the title. Well, Dean was the one I trusted to answer that critical question. One day, I found myself alone with him in the "Hospital from Hell," and I was determined to ask him how many then and there. Painful as it was to speak, I leapt right into it. I managed to slowly croak out to him every single detail of my horrible experience at that hospital. And how hurt and depressed I was as a result. I ashamedly told him I had given up. I was done. Finished fighting. Exhausted, I took a few moments to regain my strength to ask him the crucial question, "How many patches?"

I'll never forget what happened next. Before I could blurt it out, he sat down next to me and put his hand on my arm...just like Dr. Putnam and the angelic oncology nurses in the infusion center. He lowered his head, raised it, and apologized to me. "Lee, I'm so, so sorry," he said. "What you've experienced is horrible. It's inexcusable, and as a doctor, I'm appalled that this lack of compassion is happening more and more in modern medicine. So please accept my profoundest apology."

Dean hadn't done anything to me. He wasn't one of the HCPs who treated me with so little compassion in the hospital. He had never harmed or hurt me. And yet, his heartfelt apology stopped me in my tracks. This was the intimacy, the comfort and connection I had craved while I was hospitalized and hadn't gotten even a whiff of.

"I completely understand why you feel the way you feel, and I would have felt exactly the same! But," and he paused, "may I make a suggestion?" He politely asked my permission! I nodded, overwhelmed by his show of respect and the fact that he hadn't shamed me for being a guy, a man, and being a quitter. He continued, "What you didn't get from your doctors and nurses was compassion, and a lack of compassion is happening more and more in healthcare. As we get more technology, AI, medicines, more complicated machines, processes, and procedures, people forget that providing moment-to-moment compassion is absolutely critical to the best outcomes."

When I began treatment, no one had ever talked to me about my psychosocial, mental, emotional, and spiritual needs. (And gee, what a life changer that would have been if anyone had.) I had never really heard the word "compassion" used in the context of healthcare before. What did he mean, I hadn't gotten any?

"How about this?" he continued. "You're a perpetual patient. You know what compassionate patient care is—the best and the worst—better than anyone. You're a C-Level exec and you know that every business, including healthcare, has to make a profit. You're a customer service expert, and on a business level, patient care is, after all, 'customer service.' You're a good speaker, and if you survive and can speak … a cancer survivor, so people will listen to you. Instead of giving up, how about you fight and live? And if you survive, how about you start a movement or something. How about you spend the rest of your life doing something to reverse this lack of compassion that's becoming an epidemic in American medicine today?"

In that moment, that one simple second, I came alive again. My life could have real meaning and purpose. I could have value and worth to patients and HCPs. In that moment, I felt his compassion. I felt seen, heard, and respected. In that moment, I felt comforted. It was every bit as crucial to me being alive today as my physical treatment, and one thousand times more comforting. In that moment, I felt love—and that love turned me back into a living, breathing, human being. Yup. Now that I look back on it, what I felt from my dear, devoted wife Erica, Drs. Ashley, Putnam, Gabayans, my oncology nurses, radiation therapist, and countless others in my life who have treated me, was love. Love. Love.

Not surprisingly, a similar experience happened to the esteemed Kenneth Schwartz, former Secretary of Human Services for the state of Massachusetts under former Presidential Candidate Michael Dukakis. Schwartz later founded the Schwartz Center for Compassionate Healthcare as related in *Compassionomics*:

Kenneth B. Schwartz was a special person. In fact, without ever knowing it or ever intending to, he started a movement. After receiving a diagnosis of advanced lung cancer in November 1994, this 40-year-old, non-smoking, health care attorney with a wife and two-year-old son could have faced his diagnosis with bitterness or anger. Instead,

he did something truly extraordinary—
something that continues to echo throughout hospitals and health systems across the
country and has impacted innumerable lives
25 years later. It all started with an observa-
tion that he made. Then he wrote about it in
a Boston Globe Magazine article, entitled "A
Patient's Story." He observed that, as harrow-
ing as his ordeal was, it was also punctuated
by moments of exquisite compassion from
his health care providers. He was struck by
how that compassionate care could transform his experience and actually alleviate
his suffering. As he wrote in that Boston
Globe Magazine article, compassion makes
"the unbearable bearable." He described
his caregivers as people who willingly and
intentionally crossed the usual professional
barrier between health care provider and
patient (he called it the professional "rubi-
con") so they could know Schwartz as a person. They took a personal interest in him. He
also spoke of one physician scientist, Dr. Kurt
Isselbacher, who was a renowned expert
in clinical trials and director of the cancer
center at Massachusetts General Hospital.
Isselbacher was helping Schwartz navigate
which experimental therapy might be the
best to try in order to extend his life. He was
a famous researcher, but he also cared about

Schwartz and touched him with great compassion and gave him hope. Not false hope, mind you, but real hope. The kind of hope that came from Isselbacher's real experience on the cutting edge of treating cancer.

Call it love or call it compassion or call it comfort—they're all the same. They're why I'm alive today. It's why I created the CARE Effect Movement. It's why I have the privilege of spending my days traveling and spreading the word about the importance—no, the necessity—of providing compassion for patients, healthcare professionals, colleagues, friends, family, strangers, *everyone*, everywhere I go. True joy comes from fulfilling one's purpose in this life. All I have to say about that is that neither my time as a professional athlete, producing TV shows, raising tens of millions of dollars for a national charity, owning and developing movie studios, nor any other "work" I've ever done was ever remotely this fulfilling and joyous.

According to the World Health Organization (WHO) compassionate attention to the psychosocial needs of every cancer patient is "integral," not optional, to their treatment. That said, I'm certain that it's fair to say that if compassion is that powerful of a healing agent for cancer patients, it must be equally powerful for every other type of patient malady or injury. Who you are is what you leave behind. You want to leave a legacy? Leave love.

CHAPTER 5

"Love and compassion are necessities, not luxuries. Without them, humanity cannot survive."

—Dalai Lama XIV

When I first decided to take Dr. Edell's suggestion and founded the CARE Effect Movement, I had to do a lot of research to learn about the role of compassion in healthcare. For me, the first thing was to come up with a simple, clear, memorable definition of the word. As it turned out, there were thousands of peer-reviewed articles with substantiating evidence to support an irrefutable link between compassion and healing. And I studied a ton of them.

One of the first things I learned was that Charles Darwin, of Theory of Evolution fame, coined a lot more than the concept of "survival of the fittest." Darwin also believed that compassion was totally ingrained into the DNA of the human race, to the point that our species developing the ability to feel and express compassion is intrinsically linked with our continued evolution and survival as a species.

According to Darwin, the communities with the greatest compassion for others would "flourish the best and rear the greatest number of offspring." In short, the body of scientific evidence supports that compassion actually protects the species. This makes sense: the hunter that shared his extra carnings with those in need could count on others to do the same when he needed help in the future. It was the other-focused, more compassionate humans that were the ones that survived to pass on their genes. At a very basic level, research supports that compassion is something intrinsic to the human condition. For example, studies show that infants will resonate with the cries of others in distress and that toddlers are naturally inclined to altruistically help others. There is a general consensus among scientists that compassion for others is, in fact, evolutionary.[5]

A study conducted by the Cancer Care Research Professorship from the Faculty of Nursing at the

---

5 Compassionomics: The Revolutionary Scientific Evidence that Caring Makes a Difference, Stephen Trzeciak, Anthony Mazzarelli. 2018.

University of Calgary analyzed 36,637 research records of other studies addressing the role of compassion in healthcare, only to find that less than a third of the studies included patients and that only eight of the nearly 37,000 aimed to improve compassionate care in healthcare professionals. Unfortunately, this made my research exceptionally difficult. As I worked to find a scientific case for compassionate, patient-centered healthcare, I had no way of narrowing down the studies that included those patients, nor of finding the needles in the haystack that addressed how compassionate care could benefit healthcare professionals as well.

Since then, my research has become a whole lot easier. Now, concerns about subpar patient care and a lack of compassion in medical fields have led to a myriad of peer-reviewed scientific studies and thousands of additional articles from reputable sources on a subject that only a few years ago was rarely even discussed. Remember what I said about being a lifelong patient? I didn't realize how much receiving compassionate care from healthcare professionals meant until it was taken away from me in that "Hospital from Hell." When my doctors and nurses treated me with care and compassion, I felt like I wasn't going through this alone, like I was with people who really gave a crap about *me*. I wasn't just someone paying their bills.

Another segment from *Compassionomics* emphasizes the cruciality of compassionate care in each and every patient interaction—not just the most dire:

A missed opportunity for compassion can change the trajectory of one's life forever. And it's not just suicide where providers can save a life. Missed opportunities for compassionate care are also common for patients suffering during the most severe physical health crises. This is not opinion; these are the scientific data. Consider this shocking example from a rigorously conducted Johns Hopkins study: Trained observers set about measuring health care providers' verbal and non-verbal communications in the intensive care unit (ICU). In fully 74 percent of the interactions in the ICU, researchers found that the health care providers showed no compassion for patients or families (i.e., zero compassionate behaviors.

Boy, does that ever sound like my "Hospital from Hell!" As patients, we want—make that need—our providers to consistently show that they care by looking out for us. By paying attention to us and *our* needs—not theirs. That's the gift.

So when a patient is treated in a compassionate environment, they receive a myriad of measurable mental, physical, and emotional benefits. But that's not a surprise to us, right? Isn't that what providing kind, caring bedside manner is all about?

Okay. But did you also know that when healthcare providers work in a compassionate environment—that is to say, in a workplace where they are treated with the same kindness, hospitality, respect, generosity, understanding, and appreciation as is given to their patients—providers get a slew of great benefits, too?

Healthcare professionals working in compassionate workplaces have reported increased satisfaction with their jobs, less anxiety, and a lower chance of developing depression, lowered fatigue, and less of a chance of burnout, the numbers for which have increased dramatically since the additional stress and pressure of COVID-19 arrived.

> Compassion also seems to prevent doctor burnout—a condition that affects almost half of U.S. physicians. Medical schools often warn students not to get too close to patients, because too much exposure to human suffering is likely to lead to exhaustion, Trzeciak says. But the opposite appears to be true: Evidence shows that connecting with patients makes physicians happier and more fulfilled.

We've always heard that burnout crushes compassion. It's probably more likely that those people with low compassion, those are the ones that are predisposed to burnout," Trzeciak said. "That human connection—and specifically a compassionate connection—can actually build resilience and resistance to burnout.[6]

Think about it. It makes perfect sense; when you feel seen, heard, appreciated, and happier at work, you feel happier everywhere else, too—which, because compassionate care leads to faster healing, means *you'll* also experience better physical and mental health as well.

But wait! There's more! Because fostering a compassionate environment benefits patients and providers alike, medical institutions that make compassionate, patient-centered care an "integral," top priority of their culture for patients *and* providers, have lower turnover, higher patient retention, fewer medical errors, fewer lawsuits, increased employee productivity, and a more profitable bottom line due to higher HCAHP (Hospital Consumer Assessment of Healthcare Providers & Systems) scores and resultant higher Medicare reimbursements, meaning

---

6   Ritchie, L. C. (2019, April 26). Does Taking Time For Compassion Make Doctors Better At Their Jobs? Retrieved from https://www.npr.org/sections/health-shots/2019/04/26/717272708/does-taking-time-for-compassion-make-doctors-better-at-their-jobs

that healthcare professionals have greater job security because their workplaces are not, like many others these days, in dire financial straits.

The number one determining factor in whether or not a patient gives a higher HCAHP score is if they're cared for with compassion while they're being treated. Duh! It's whether or not their caregivers—in every function—work in a compassionate environment. And who is responsible for that?

You are. Period. They're also *your* exhausted, hurting, suffering colleagues, and how you treat them is how they'll treat the rest of the world—including you, your patients, and colleagues.

The Beryl Institute states accurately that patient experience is the "sum of all interactions" while being treated—worst and best.[7] Some people may say their care was "OK," but the majority asked have a very strong opinion one way or the other. However, a patient or a customer's experience is disproportionately influenced as the result of one "deep" experience—and that experience will be highly positive or negative. Yes, a patient's experience is an amalgamation of all their interactions from the moment they call to make an appointment, but that one experience will stay with them—and sometimes their providers—for the rest of their lives. Not the

---

7   What is Patient Experience? (n.d.). Retrieved June 24, 2019, from https://www.theberylinstitute.org/page/DefiningPatientExp

jabs, cuts, and pain, but the comfort of knowing that someone they trust, who they know truly cares, is on their side and there for them when they need it the most. Wow! That's a gift of the highest order … a true blessing.

Remember being the person to provide that experience? Isn't that a gift for you both? How good does that feel for you? Heavenly, right?

CHAPTER 6

"Too often we underestimate the power of a
touch, a smile, a kind word, a listening ear,
an honest compliment, or the smallest act
of caring, all of which have the potential to
turn a life around."

—Leo Buscaglia

Imagine you're at work and you're told that a truly
mentally ill person is going to be brought into the
room. Upon entry, that person begins to threaten
and verbally attack you. Do you take it personally?

No, right? Why? Because you understand that
they're mentally challenged and not fully aware or
in control of their actions. Well, sometimes when
we're sick or injured, we're all more than a little off
too. And sometimes, when providing care for someone who's sick, you probably have found yourself a
little crazed, too.

The simple fact of the matter is that people who
hurt people are always, always experiencing enormous mental, physical, emotional, and/or spiritual

pain. That doesn't excuse their hurtful behavior, but it does make it understandable, and with understanding comes empathy; and often, empathy—well, it turns into compassion. Aha!

If you want to give your very best, compassionate self to someone in pain, it's not a choice. You must not take your pain out on others. We *all* have pain. But if you're in healthcare, you have a moral imperative to never take it out on your patients or your colleagues. Period.

Fortunately, though often painfully, compassion requires that we look very deeply inside ourselves, into our deepest pain and do whatever it takes to prevent ourselves from taking that pain out on vulnerable patients or on colleagues who will then take it out on their patients or colleagues. Compassion expressed outwardly and pain expressed outwardly are both "catching." It's scientifically proven that more often than not, people given kindness pass it on to others—and people treated hurtfully do too!

If you were lucky when you were hurt as a kid, you had understanding guardians who weren't upset when you screamed and cried and punished you somehow for it. They felt compassion for you and gave you the hug and kiss and comfort you so desperately needed. That's what we patients are begging for. It sounds easy enough. Just one problem—it's hard to be a comfort when you yourself are in pain and in need of comfort.

Yes, there is a massive crisis in medicine, for patients and our country. Too many people can't afford medical treatment because of its cost, and for those who can, the cost often leaves them destitute or among the 48 percent of Americans who file for bankruptcy from these healthcare related costs. For those who can't afford it—well, they just get sicker, suffer, and die. A tragedy in the richest country in the world and the antithesis of compassion.

But even for those who can afford to get treated, there is another huge problem. That is, once they're getting their treatment, they are highly likely *not* to be treated in a kind, caring, and compassionate environment, which you'll recall, has been scientifically proven to be "integral" to the best possible outcomes for patients by the World Health Organization.

Even worse, nearly 50 percent of Americans believe that neither their healthcare system—nor their practitioners—have the slightest bit of compassion! And that means that 50 percent of America's patients are being denied the compassionate care deemed "integral" or essential to the best possible outcomes!

In other words, a critical component of their treatment, in some cases the difference between life and death, is being denied to them.

And that is a clear violation of Hippocrates's age-old healthcare professional promise to "first do no harm."

When I made the decision to fight and live, things didn't magically come together for me. I was still incredibly sick and in astounding physical pain that drove me to the edge of sanity on a daily basis. Regardless, I had to get clear on what my life's mission was going to manifest as, and I'm ashamed to admit that at first, I thought that meant identifying monsters like the ones who had so poorly cared for me at the "Hospital from Hell" and vengefully force them out of medicine. I had no idea how to do that, but I was determined to orchestrate the dismissal of every compassionless healthcare provider in America. Seriously! I wasn't angry—I was raging.

Luckily for those providers—and, ultimately, for me—there wasn't a lot I could do while still so sick and weak. I remembered that when Dr. Edell had so lovingly comforted me, he'd used the word "compassion" and said it had been denied to me. I started to look past the dictionary definition of the word and try to find out what the heck it was and why he thought it was so important. What was the big deal?

At the time, I couldn't have defined compassion for you if you'd offered me a new thumb. Not a clue. I'd have probably defined empathy instead, as most people do, the willingness to feel the pain of others. I had no sense of the value for patients or providers or anyone else. But as I began to read what evidence was available, I was astounded at the value for both. I mean, who knew? Only with the release of the recent *Compassionomics* book have those studies been tallied—and they are nothing short of amazing!

So with all of this empirical evidence, why would anybody in healthcare fail to engage with patients in any manner other than spectacularly wonderfully? Why wouldn't every patient in the world have the most compassionate care possible? I couldn't understand. Weirder still, I knew where people can be almost 100 percent certain to experience compassion when they're suffering. In hospice. What? We reserve our greatest expressions of kindness and compassion until someone is close to death? So we don't deserve it until then, despite the empirical benefits that increase the chances of a cure? How is that right?

It took a long time, but I eventually found a major contributor to those questions— healthcare professional burnout.

> Research shows there has been an erosion of the relationship between those who provide health care and the patients they treat, and specifically an erosion of compassion. Nearly half of Americans believe the U.S. health-care system and health-care providers are not compassionate, one survey found. Numerous studies have reported that physicians miss the majority of opportunities to respond to patients with compassion. Research on the burnout epidemic in health

care finds that 35 percent of physicians are so burned out that they have an inability to make a personal connection with patients. This can result in callous or uncaring behavior.[8]

An "inability!" And it's not just doctors. It's *everyone* who works in healthcare. Doctors, nurses, administrators, everyone. Even if they were aware of their state, which is unlikely when burned out, they'd be unable to provide compassion under any circumstances. Zero. And that's a killer of both HCPs *and* patients. Forget the bottom line—but there, too.

From my perpetual patient's perspective, this is *the* biggest, most disturbing statistic in healthcare. It means that 50 percent of American patients are not being treated compassionately. That means they're not even getting adequate medical treatment, let alone optimal. And, that's why I'm doing what I'm doing.

It's worth noting that burnout isn't the only answer for the questions posed above, but it is a

---

8 Trzeciak, S., & Mazzarelli, A. (2019, May 12). For patients, a caregiver's compassion is essential. Retrieved from https://www.washingtonpost.com/national/health-science/for-patients-a-caregivers-compassion-is-essential/2019/05/10/6aa513ce-6b5 8-11e9-8f44-e8d8bb1df986_story.html?utm_term=. d262d49c41f7

primary one, and burnout is becoming responsible for new issues stemming from less-than- compassionate care every day.

Ian MacLaren had it right when he said, "Be kind, for everyone you meet is fighting a hard battle."

Everyone, in healthcare and otherwise, if they were honest, sat down and really thought about it, has a lot of pain from the myriad of sad, disappointing, upsetting, heartbreaking, and discouraging events in their present or past. And, unless effectively dealt with and released, with that pain comes suffering.

In terms of personality types, a large percentage of healthcare providers are people-pleasers by nature—not in a bad way. It's just how they operate. Why else would anyone elect to work at a hospital or in a medical practice? Neither is it about "hats and horns" as my former business partner used to say. No one goes to hospitals for fun. People go because they are in pain, either personally or in pain for someone they know and love. And so are their families and friends, because their family members and friends are in pain, too.

And yet healthcare providers go there willingly, happily, devotedly, despite all of that. Day after day, week after week, year after year. Not because it's easy, but because it's brutally hard and someone has to do it, and that someone is them! It's just who they are and it's what drives them. It's not a job. It's their calling, their mission, their purpose in life.

But the fact is, you can never heal everybody. So our doctors and nurses and other HCPs work and work and work and too often don't allow themselves to consider that their own health and well-being should take priority over that of their patients and colleagues so they're healthy and able to be their most competent and compassionate selves when we patients need it the most.

It seems noble, and to a point, it is. But if it leads to burnout, it's actually harmful to everybody. Patients, colleagues, the bottom line, and themselves.

In 2019, the World Health Organization codified burnout as a legitimate medical diagnosis, meaning that doctors can now diagnose someone with burnout if they meet a list of common symptoms. It's a move that comes better late than never in a profession that ranks higher than any other for suicide—doctors![9]

I often think about the ways in which this whole experience has come full circle for me, from burnout back to brilliance. When I realized that burnout is a major statistical issue in healthcare, I took a look at a list of the qualities of someone with burnout. They included, among others, the following: feelings of

---

9   Anderson, P. (2018, May 08). Doctors' Suicide Rate Highest of Any Profession. Retrieved from https://www.webmd.com/mental-health/news/20180508/doctors-suicide-rate-highest-of-any-profession#1

energy depletion or exhaustion; increased mental distance from one's job, or feelings of negativism or cynicism related to one's job; reduced efficiency in a professional capacity;[10] excessive stress; fatigue; insomnia; sadness, anger, irritability, impatience; and vulnerability to illnesses.[11] How would you like to be cared for by someone exhibiting those qualities? Trust me. I have, and you don't want to.

The list went on. The simple fact is that hurt people hurt people, to be quite frank, and that's when I realized—*I* was totally burned out when I was diagnosed with cancer. I mean, I fit every criterion, and even though I thought I was being diligent and hardworking and trying to save myself and everyone

---

10 QD85 Burn-out. (n.d.). Retrieved from https://icd. who.int/browse11/l-m/en#/http://id.who.int/icd/ entity/129180281 Burn-out is a syndrome conceptualized as resulting from chronic workplace stress that has not been successfully managed. It is characterized by three dimensions: 1) feelings of energy depletion or exhaustion; 2) increased mental distance from one's job, or feelings of negativism or cynicism related to one's job; and 3) reduced professional efficacy. Burn-out refers specifically to phenomena in the occupational context and should not be applied to describe experiences in other areas of life.

11 Know the signs of job burnout. (2018, November 21). Retrieved from https://www.mayoclinic.org/ healthy-lifestyle/adult-health/in-depth/burnout/ art-20046642

around me, I was actually kind of a jerk to most everyone—loved ones, friends, colleagues, family. Everyone! Why? Because I was in misery—mentally, emotionally, physically, romantically, financially, professionally. I didn't even know it or deal with it in a healthy way.

I knew then that the people who treated me so poorly in that hospital didn't deserve to be punished, nor did any of the millions of other burned-out medical professionals like them. They needed to be held responsible, but what they needed most of all was understanding and compassion and help healing.

Now that I realized I had experienced and survived burnout myself, it was infinitely easier for me not to accept but to understand how it must feel to have so much life-saving and life-giving responsibility on one's shoulders every day, with no end in sight. I developed a level of empathy that I would have thought impossible mere months earlier. I realized that healthcare professionals are far too often literally killing themselves on my behalf and on the behalf of their patients, that they're trying their best, and in that moment, I resolved to see if I couldn't help rather than punish them.

Hurt people, hurt people. More violence, more guns, more weapons isn't going to solve anything, as we're seeing now following the horrific death of George Floyd and the subsequent violence and looting. That just deepens the chasm between us and them. The only solution is to listen deeply to their stories, try to understand where their pain comes from—see if your empathy, your understanding doesn't sometimes turn into a calm compassion and a desire to right the wrongs that resulted in that tragedy with both sides the better for it. The one who understands and empathizes and helps the other heal as the result of that compassionate act. Compassion is the answer. To all the pain—old and new—we all feel today. Period. And how you express it, that's up to you. But it starts and ends with simple human kindness for one's self and then one's fellow human beings.

Speaking to healthcare professionals around the world has been a deeply cathartic process for me. As I express my gratitude to doctors and nurses and other HCPs around the world, as well as my interest in helping them maintain or regain their health, they've expressed their gratitude back to me.

I go out and speak to share the benefit of my experience, and hopefully to save patients and healthcare providers alike from the pain that I endured. But it's when the incredible audiences with whom I've had the great good fortune to interact express their gratitude and compassion back to me, then it gives me strength. When my throat is aching, when I'm exhausted and experiencing my never-ending cancer treatment side effects—it inspires me to get up in the morning and do it again. If you're kind and compassionate to your colleagues, they're way more likely to be kind and compassionate to their other colleagues and we patients. I've felt what it's like to be appreciated. The conversations I've had with grateful audiences, people's feedback, gave me a sense of value and self-worth to know that I could help heal them.

Those audiences didn't treat me. They didn't cure me. It was their feedback that I made a difference in their lives that comforted and helped heal me. That's the feeling you get when you give compassion to patients or anyone else. You know you made a material difference in the quality of their life. So when I say it's a big deal, it's a huge deal. But someone's gotta be the first one to do it! Turns out, compassion is catching. Like a positive virus. Yup! Who knew? It's been a deeply healing process for me to be able to talk about my failures, to be able to talk about my weaknesses, my hurtful expressions of anger and rage at God and cancer and the world. It wasn't so long ago that I was behaving like a real jerk, and I didn't even know it. It stands to reason that the vast majority of burned-out healthcare providers might not know it, either. Given their life's purpose, if they did, I'd bet that the vast majority of them would take the steps to heal themselves immediately.

Consider the following:

Compelling data on the health benefits of interpersonal relationships can be traced back decades. In 1988 researchers from the University of Michigan published a landmark paper entitled "Social Relationships and Health" in the prestigious journal *Science*. They analyzed the available evidence from population-based studies and concluded that, after taking into account people's baseline health status, there was an increased risk of death among persons who have a low quantity (or low quality) of personal relationships. They also concluded that social isolation is a major risk factor for dying from a wide variety of causes: "Social relationships, or the relative lack thereof, constitute a major risk factor for health– rivaling the effect of well-established health risk factors such as cigarette smoking, blood pressure, blood lipids (cholesterol), obesity and physical activity.[12]

For the first time, it was beginning to become clear: loneliness kills. Put another way by a scientist who studies emotions, "Such an existence is too expensive to bear. When launching a life raft, the prudent survivalist will not toss food overboard while retaining the deck furniture. If somebody must jettison a part of life, time with a mate should

---

12 "Social Relationships and Health," James S. House, Karl R. Landis, August 1988.

be last on the list: [one] needs that connection to live."[13]

Compassion is both life-saving and life-changing. Will every compassionate act save a life? No. But are you willing to withhold your compassion from someone in pain only to find they'd ended their lives as a result? Of course not. It's just not who you really are.

Mandy Hale perhaps said it best. She said, "It's not selfish to love yourself, take care of yourself, and to make your happiness a priority. It's a necessity." I couldn't have said it better myself.

I've always had a bad habit of putting everyone else's needs before mine. I was once a habitual people-pleaser in the worst possible way. When I was a kid, I was always taught that doing kind things for myself was selfish, narcissistic, and self-centered. As a result, I've spent most of my life running myself ragged, taking care of everyone else's needs before my own. And what did that get me? Mental, physical, emotional, and spiritual burnout, which I took out on … everyone. Especially those closest to me. I was stressed to the max and deeply depressed, battling everything from lawsuits against my former partners to multiple deaths in our family. My mother had a variety of age-related health issues, including

13 Compassionomics: The Revolutionary Scientific Evidence that Caring Makes a Difference, Stephen Trzeciak, Anthony Mazzarelli. 2018.

a broken hip just a week after I began cancer treatment. In the deepest throes of my depression, I felt completely and utterly emotionally numb.

I learned too late that in addition to making it impossible to be compassionate to others, burnout weakens one's immune system. It was while I was totally burned-out that I contracted Stage III+ throat cancer. Coincidence? I don't think so.

Here's what I've learned. Endlessly doing for others without doing for oneself what is necessary to be healthy and happy is a disaster for everyone in your life, starting with you! You can't give what you haven't got. Be loving to yourself for the sake of your family, friends, colleagues, and hospital patients. But mostly, be loving to yourself for your own sake. You deserve it and nothing less!

If you are lucky enough to realize before it's too late that you are totally burned-out, or rapidly approaching it, please, please get professional help. Fast. Trust me. You don't want to do it on your own. I know that admitting to being burned-out can really, really hurt. But, if you don't effectively deal with it and heal, it will deeply harm you and everyone you come in contact with.

That said, if you find yourself experiencing some of the symptoms of early burn-out, allow me to share with you some of my favorite little tips and tricks for self-care that I discovered during my recovery from burnout:

1. Tell everyone you're going out of town but stay home instead. Turn off your phone, don't check your email, and stay the heck away from your computer. Spend the day enjoying 100 percent "you" time.

2. Go on the Groupon or Living Social websites to get a great deal on a massage, then go get one.

3. Light some candles, turn off the lights, and take a hot shower or bath. Then pour yourself a glass of wine, or schnapps, or beer, and play some relaxing music.

4. Sit on a beach or at a park and watch the sun go down.

5. Buy and read a trashy celebrity magazine. Update yourself on the Kardashians. You know you want to.

6. Go to a midday matinee movie, buy a big, big bag of popcorn—with butter—and a guilty-pleasure drink, lean back, and enjoy yourself. You'll probably have the theater all to yourself. Fall asleep if the mood strikes you. Snore if you like.

7. Put your pajamas on and kick your feet up. Relax, order in, put on your favorite TV series and binge a little. Nah, binge a lot. And, hey, let yourself fall asleep if you want to.

8. Buy yourself a fresh bouquet of flowers to smell and see in your home.

9. Get your filthy car detailed at a great car wash.

10. Find the coziest corner at the coffee shop, order a latte, and read half a trashy novel without interruption.

Because of my new life "purpose," I've gotten to spend many of my days wandering from floor to floor at the superb UCLA Ronald Reagan Hospital, where I've been a patient for over sixty-five years, working with patients, doctors, nurses, medical and nursing students, and administrators.

At every turn, I see patients and HCPs in great pain, fear clouding their eyes. I watch family members file out of the hospital with small bags filled with the personal effects of a loved one they've just lost, filled with grief and heartbroken sorrow.

One day, I sat next to a fellow in the cafeteria about to check into the hospital for some sort of surgery who was "getting his estate in order," just in case. I saw cancer patients who looked just like I once had: skinny, bald, nauseated, depressed, feeling ugly and despondent. I watched people angry as all heck, taking it out on people like you who had nothing to do with why they were angry.

People work hard to never go to the hospital. But you do willingly, with love, every single day. Out of your devotion to treat, cure, and comfort your fellow human beings when they need your skills more than ever.

I have one word for you. Bravo. You are my heroes!

You are brave. You are tough. You have hearts bigger than anyone. You are my heroes, and the heroes of every patient, whether they tell you or not. I salute you; I am honored to know you, and I am deeply, deeply inspired by your humanity and expressions of compassion. I'm almost certain you don't receive enough praise for what you do. Letting yourself be proud of who you are and the work you do is just as much a part of self-care as any tip or trick I could offer.

To me, the idea of self-care can be summarized by one semi-profound Secret of the Universe: "Eat Dessert First."

If I've learned anything from all of my most painful life experiences, getting older, and watching some dear people leave this earth, it is this:

Figure out what gives you pleasure, then do it. Now. Often. Not in a few days, weeks, months, or years. Why? Because there is no guarantee that you'll have even one more day, week, month, or year. I know you think you'll live for years and years to come. And, while I hope so, the honest answer is that we can't guarantee such things. I went to see my ENT seemingly healthy as all heck about some allergies and came out with a cancer diagnosis that almost killed me and nearly destroyed my life.

So, just to make sure you have no regrets, start by eating dessert first. People say, "Leave the best for last," to which I say, horse manure. Clearly, they've never had a life-threatening disease or injury.

So get that foot rub, take that vacation, sleep an extra fifteen minutes, take an afternoon off and just hang, treat your little niece to lunch, and "Eat Dessert First."

Because you can. Because you must!

Finally, I'd be remiss not to mention one of the simplest things a person can do to revive and renew themselves mentally, physically, and emotionally: meditate. The only difference between meditating today and thousands of years ago is that the benefits are now scientifically proven.

1. It makes you healthier.
2. It makes you happier.
3. It improves your social life.
4. It increases your self-control.
5. It changes your brain for the better.
6. It improves your productivity.
7. It makes you wiser.

And, it's incredibly simple to do. Sit comfortably upright, close your eyes, and breathe. That's it. If I can do it, so can you! For how long? As long as you have. One minute. Ten. Thirty. An hour. You choose. Every little bit helps.

So, here is the question. Knowing scientifically that your compassion can improve both the recipient and giver's ability to heal, lessen pain, improve immune function, and just plain make you feel "better," what could possibly stop you? Why would you not give it to everyone, including yourself, all the time?

You are a healer. You have a power that modern medicine cannot and never will replicate. You have the gift of compassion that if bestowed improves the lives of everyone involved in the equation. To paraphrase Yoda, you do or you don't. There is no "try."

As famed musician and meditator Ravi Shankar once said, "The quality of our life depends on the quality of our mind."

A bad day, a bad week, a bad year makes it difficult to show compassion. But easy or difficult, isn't that what you got into medicine to do in the first place? And, if you don't give your compassion away freely, isn't that a rejection of the most important values that you hold dearest?

It is. And that's not you. You are better and bigger than that. You have chosen a life of service. Your compassionate heart is the one gift that only *you* can give.

So, be yourself. Your best self. Be the best healer you were born to be. Small, kind, caring, thoughtful, and compassionate acts could mean the difference between life and death for you, your colleagues, and your patients. Give freely, no matter what.

I'm counting on you. And, frankly, so is the world.

CHAPTER 7

"No act of kindness, no matter how small, is
ever wasted."

—Aesop

A few years ago, I caught a segment on *CBS News
Sunday Morning* about a young man who had
experienced childhood obesity, a family torn apart
by drugs, and homelessness all before he reached
high school. With the loving kindness and compassionate ears of his brother, aunt, and a gentle-
man who adopted him in the sixth grade, he lost
weight, found a stable home, and won Indiana's
Mr. Basketball award, all in the same year. They
didn't give him money. They didn't provide him
with material luxuries. They provided love and compassion. He earned a 3.3 GPA, was scouted by several
colleges, wound up playing for Purdue, then the
NBA. What a gift for them all.

In healthcare, how many kids—heck, how
many people—do you see in a day that you could
be a model for? Your mission in life is to treat

people compassionately because they matter, and you believe in their importance as humans—no matter what extenuating circumstances you or they may be facing.

Remember that thing I said about compassion being catching? Did you know that it, too, has been scientifically proven? Yup, compassion is catching just like a virus, but in a good way. There have been numerous experiments conducted on toll bridges and elsewhere where one person intentionally pays for themselves *and* the person behind them. Know what happens?

You got it. That person who just got the freebie pays for the person behind them and that keeps happening again and again for hours on end. When you get compassion, you naturally want to pass it onward. It's how we are genetically created. It's in our genes.

I've had the immense pleasure to see that in action time and again, and the more the CARE Effect Movement grows, the more aware I become of everyday acts of kindness and compassion and the opportunities to provide them that I'd likely never have seen before.

One morning, when I arrived at UCLA to consult with their Enrollment Management Department during a multiyear effort to inspire and support their staff in being more kind, caring, and compassionate with applicants and their families, a homeless woman, no shoes, nose bloodied, dirty, shivering, was sitting outside my client's office.

I saw her before I even got out of the car. Now, I just can't pass by people like that and pretend I don't see them. So, I gathered up all the spare change I keep in the car for parking meters, added a couple of dollar bills and gave them to her.

As you might well imagine, she was very grateful. But this is where the story gets interesting. When I spoke with her, I saw that she was shivering and really needed a warm coat. So I went into the building and asked one of the staff if they had a lost-and-found and if so, was there perhaps a coat that had been there forever—this homeless woman needed it. The receptionist said there was nothing in the lost-and-found, but that she, personally, had an extra coat which she was happy to give to the poor freezing woman.

But wait—it gets better. Some other staff members caught wind of what was happening, and guess what? They gathered up a bunch of food and a box of much-needed Kleenex and gave that to her, as well.

Then we noticed that she had no shoes. I asked a woman in my meeting where I could buy her a pair on campus. She then told me that she kept a pair of tennis shoes for emergencies that were—if you can believe it—size seven and a half, exactly that woman's shoe size, which we gave to her immediately after our meeting.

This wonderfully heartening day for all of us involved calls to mind a "fascinating randomized controlled trial" conducted by the University of Toronto in 1995.

Researchers tested if especially compassionate care for homeless patients in the emergency department would affect their subsequent use of emergency services. They randomized 133 homeless patients arriving in the emergency department with no identifiable diagnosis into two groups: one group was assigned to receive extra compassionate care from a trained volunteer (a person whose only job was to treat the homeless patients with extra compassion) in addition to usual care from the emergency department staff. The other group was assigned to usual care only. They tested the association between extra compassion and return visits to the emergency department over the next thirty days. And what did they find out? Compared to usual care, randomization to extra compassion reduced subsequent emergency department visits by homeless patients by 33 percent. These results are based on a randomized trial with a rigorous experimental design. So they are based on science; not a set of beliefs or opinions.[14]

---

14 Compassionomics: The Revolutionary Scientific Evidence that Caring Makes a Difference, Stephen Trzeciak, Anthony Mazzarelli. 2018.

One day, I promise you—if you haven't already, or if you have—you'll be in a situation where you desperately want your nurse, doctor, housekeeper, food service professionals, and everyone else around you to give you the kindness and compassion you really need. So remember, compassion and its results are catching. One day I promise you'll crave it, and won't you be relieved to know that you get what you give. Give compassion—get compassion. Simple. Not easy. But you knew that. That's why you took the job. You knew you were up to the challenge, right?

That is how compassion works. All you have to do is start the ball rolling with your one more compassionate act today. The rest is magic.

CHAPTER 8

"More smiling, less worrying. More compassion, less judgment. More blessed, less stressed. More love, less hate."

—Roy T. Bennett

The blessings of cancer? Seriously!

I gotta tell you, it was a couple years before I saw it as a blessing in even the most minute way. It was a terrible curse as far as I was concerned, and I was furious about it. Raving mad. Throughout my treatment and for many months after, I was so filled with rage that if God Himself had walked in the room I'd have fought him.

I had many angry conversations with God during this time. *God, let me see if I understand this. You created the universe and everything in it. You're all-powerful. You own, and control, all creation. So why did you give me cancer? Did I deserve it? Is this punishment? And if so, for what? Because if this is some kind of karmic retribution, I know some people who should have had cancer nine times before me.*

I learned a lot of lessons from cancer, and one of those was that I absolutely could have used a nurse or non-nurse navigator. Someone who had been through the cancer treatment process before and knew the ins and outs. My diagnosis, and all that followed, came so quickly and without warning that I felt as if my brain had exploded.

It was absolutely impossible for me to remember everything that I was being told. There was an incredible amount of information, and it kept coming, and coming, and coming to this very day.

If it wasn't with the illness, it was with the treatment, it was with the insurance, it was with the options, it was with where, it was with whom. There were a million, trillion questions. If I had had someone as my advocate, that problem would have been dissolved.

Not to say that the questions wouldn't have been any less difficult to answer, but I would have had help in answering them.

The second thing I learned is that having cancer makes a person very lonely. Because cancer itself is so scary for most people, not everyone will be thrilled to talk about it with you or even be around you while you are being treated. I totally understand and get that. What I found is that since you get isolated a lot when you're ill, it's really important not to go it alone and get help; which is to say, to put yourself in situations with fellow cancer patients, to talk about your illness in ways that you only can with fellow patients.

There is an organization called the National Cancer Support Community, which offers those exact kinds of services; and in addition to being a source of the most up-to-date cancer related information on all fronts, they offer weekly support groups with other cancer patients led by trained mental health professionals. They also offer similar groups for caregivers, as well—and trust me, my wife and I are eternally grateful for all their help to get us through it. You, and your family, and your caregivers can all take advantage of it. You can get out of the isolation that cancer puts you in and talk about it with people who really get what you're going through—your fellow cancer patients. Oh, and did I mention that it is all free? Free! You just have to ask. How cool is that in today's prohibitively expensive medical arena? The National Cancer Support Community's work literally defines compassion.

The third thing is you'll need help with the everyday stuff. You'll need help from family and friends. It is absolutely imperative, that if you're lucky enough to have a primary caregiver, that you help them get some relief from the ongoing myriad of stresses your treatment entails by getting other people involved. Simply reach out and ask them for their help. Many want to and just need to be asked. Some will say no because they literally can't handle it. and that's understandable. It's not an easy thing to handle. It is scary, for both the caregiver as well as for the patient, but if you can line up some friends who you're close to, and get the love and support from them that you need, you will both be well served.

People would always say to me when I was being treated—and please don't ever say this to a cancer patient—"You know, when one door closes, another door opens." Give me a break. I had cancer, an experience that would never truly go away. Even if it went into remission, it would impact me profoundly for the rest of my life. I didn't want to hear about doors opening or closing.

I was surviving, but I was angry, and for a long time, the anger is what kept me going. It wasn't until I realized that healthcare providers—like the ones who had so mistreated me while I was hospitalized with that septic infection—were not uncaring, but burned out from caring and giving too much, that my eyes were opened to the real issue in healthcare and things started to turn around for me.

One day, I heard somebody say that line to me, again, "When one door closes another door opens…" and then they added another that changed everything. They added, "… but people are so focused on doors that have closed that they never notice the doors that are opening." Whoa! That simple change in wording changed my whole perspective about the idea that *good* could actually come from deep pain and suffering, and I began to look for it. I was shocked by the blessings I began to see once I had that perspective.

As I mentioned before, I'd always wanted to be a doctor or nurse and help heal people. Now I get to devote myself full-time to helping heal the people who heal people. I get to play golf all over the world with people of all races, cultures, and creeds when I speak to them. I get to have the fun, at my age, of starting a new business. I get to spend time with fellow cancer survivors, celebrating the simple joy of life. What a blessing. That is an honor beyond my imagination. And my job? I get to tell stories. How cool is that?

My finances are far from stable. My love life? Virtually nonexistent. Materialistically, I have fewer belongings than ever. I'm scared every day that I'm going to relapse ... and yet I'm happier than I've ever been. Joyous, even.

So why did I get cancer? I think I might have figured it out.

When my brother-in-law told me that he understood why I was so despondent and had given up but said, "Why don't you live and become a part of the solution?" all of a sudden, he renewed my will to live and gave me a reason to do what I do. All of a sudden, for the first time in my life, I instantly realized this is why I was put on this earth. *This* is why I got cancer. My life's purpose. Everything before this had just been preparatory.

I've come to the realization that you learn things differently from a physical demonstration than from purely intellectual ones. God knew what I wanted to learn in this life. I believe that God wanted me to be a teacher—not in the religious sense, but to attempt to inspire people and to help reconnect them with their souls. And, not just healthcare professionals, everyone.

On my former path, something like what I do now would never have been conceivable, let alone possible. The more I became involved with professional sports, television, and film, the sum total of the good I was able to do for other human beings was miniscule. Not because I was a bad person, but because my businesses were the antithesis of learning to grow in empathy and compassion, and in expressing them. I worked with executives so cruel that I'd leave meetings to go to my car and cry. I worked with crooked partners who embezzled a ton from our business. God gave me the chance to get out of those situations and follow my true inclinations—to give value and service to others in a capacity that I never had before. And yes, I believe that to do that, God allowed me to get cancer.

I lost my business, my fortune, my health, my wife, my career—cancer took away everything that I had, but it led to where I am now, where I've never been so joyous.

So why did God let me get cancer? Because we had a deal that God would bring me challenges I could learn from. And what I wanted to learn from this life was to love myself and to be as loving, kind, caring, and compassionate as I possibly could, for my betterment and the betterment of the world.

While I don't believe that cancer itself is a blessing—far from it—it did bring numerous blessings to my life, the likes of which I could never previously have imagined. I was hardheaded about it for a while, but I finally saw the doors that were opening. Now I'm free.

I mean it when I say I've never been as grateful, joyous, or fulfilled as I have been in these last few years, traveling around the world to speak to healthcare providers and patients about the CARE Effect Movement and the importance of combating burnout and expressing one's innate compassion. I love seeing new places, meeting new people, and learning new things from new experiences. But what really makes it so wonderfully, beautifully satisfying to do what I do is the proof that the CARE Effect works—the reassurances from real people that I'm making a real difference in their lives.

I've got to admit, it makes me feel deeply humbled and grateful to read some of the responses people have had to my work:

> "Hearing Lee's talk should be a requirement of every medical and surgical resident. Heck, it should be a requirement of every medical professional. Period!"
> —Dr. G, UCLA Medical Center, Ronald Reagan Hospital, UCLA Medical Center

"I challenge you to listen to survivor and patient-care expert Lee Tomlinson who offers compassionate solutions that improve outcomes, incomes, healing, compliance, clinician burn-out and above all, patient satisfaction."

—Dr. Dean Edell, pioneering TV and radio medical talk show host

"Lee crushed it! His thank you at the end provoked tears and goosebumps through the room. Awesome insight. Excellent job … truly excellent."

—Jeffrey Weisgerber, marketing, oncology, TEDxLilly curator, Eli Lilly and Company

"I've lost track of how many standing ovations Lee has gotten from packed houses who instantly fall in love with him and his message. If you're looking for someone to inspire others to live and work with more compassion, look no further than "Patient Lee.'"

—Shola Richards, best-selling author and workplace positivity activist

"Lee was brilliant. My nurses were deeply moved and inspired and learned practical ways to provide even more compassionate care for their patients and—more importantly—themselves. Book him. Your nurses, your hospital and your patients will all benefit."

—Catherine Gabster, MSN, RN, CNL, CNS, Clinical Nurse Specialist at Ronald Reagan UCLA Medical Center, Ronald Reagan Hospital

Wow. Wow. But it's not my ego that's buoyed by these wonderful people and their wonderful words—it's my soul. I've devoted the rest of my life to making a measurable impact, to starting a compassionate movement. It's deeply healing to hear from people for whom I have the utmost respect, and who are under no obligation to offer such wonderful commentary on my work, offer these endorsements of their own accord and from a place of genuine gratitude.

This is, to me, qualitative evidence that the CARE Effect accomplishes much more than just buoying spirits. It has and continues to inspire people in my audiences to commit to performing intentional, compassionate actions—recorded daily—to ensure their health, happiness, and avoid "burn-out" in order to be healthy enough to present their most compassionate selves when we patients so desperately need it.

Given my health history, my age, and the fact that nearly 50 percent of Americans believe that healthcare and healthcare professionals totally lack compassion, I am even more determined to do whatever I can, as quickly as I can, to reach as many of the nearly twenty million HCPs as humanly possible before I leave this planet.

My life revolves around reaching as many healthcare professionals with my message about the *necessity* of providing compassionate care—in addition to great technically competent treatment—for patients *and* themselves to better be able to do so.

How often does God give us a second chance to stop, reflect, think, and feel in order to decide what is truly important to us as human beings? He has given us the chance to do that now. Sometimes, it's just nice to be reminded that I'm on the right path.

Epilogue

"True compassion means not only feeling another's pain, but also being motivated to help relieve it."

—Daniel Galeman

Last year, I was sitting in my oncologist's office having my semiannual checkup. After two hours of tests, I heard him unexpectedly gasp. Oh, crap. Not again. The last time I heard that sound in Dr. Putnam's office, it had not been good news.

"Lee," he said surprised, "Did you know it's been exactly five years to the day since you had your last oncology treatment? Do you know what that means?" I shook my head. Not a clue. "We're not supposed to use this word, but—statistically—it means you're cured." Wait. What? I didn't even know that that was possible! Stunned into silence, a rare occurrence for me, I returned home and told my roommate, one of the most extraordinary and compassionate women I've ever known.

Her first reaction was to literally jump for joy and say we had to celebrate! No kidding. I suggested a great dinner at the best restaurant in nearby Beverly Hills. She suggested skydiving. My first reaction? Nooooooooo! I'd just beaten cancer by an inch and now I was going to risk my life—again—and jump out of an airplane? No way. Then she asked the one question she knew would get me to go. "Are you ... afraid?" And so, at sixty-nine, I jumped out of an airplane at 13,500 feet.

There was a time when my two greatest fears were jumping out of an airplane and dying of cancer. Now, I've beaten 'em both. Woohoo!

I'm now cancer-free, and I spend my days doing work I love, with people I love, paying it forward, and even finding time for a few rounds of golf. I'm not bragging—OK, maybe a little—but I recently even "shot my age," a two under par sixty-nine, an extremely rare golf achievement that a mere 0.0000089 percent of all people who play golf (less than nine golfers per million) ever accomplish! Woohoo, life is good!

So let me say one simple thing in parting. Thank you for treating me. Thank you for curing me. But mostly, thank you for comforting me when I needed it the most. I am forever in your debt. I love you, I love you, I love you.

ACKNOWLEDGEMENTS

This book was a long, long time coming, and without the aid of so many extraordinarily smart, kind, caring, and compassionate people, it would never have come to be, and honestly, I wouldn't have been alive to write it.

I'd like to single out a few here for their contributions to my life today by nursing me back to health and thus allowing me to fulfill my new, post-cancer "life purpose" through my work with the CARE Effect Movement.

Carol and Tom Tomlinson
What can I say about my mom and dad? They made me the man I am today. Without them, I wouldn't be alive for a wide variety of reasons. My mom was the living embodiment of kindness and compassion for me and everyone else she came in contact with throughout her brilliantly artistic, creative, and loving ninety-three-year life. In the dictionary under perseverance and hard work is a picture of my dad. When push came to shove in the darkest hours of

my cancer treatment and since, it was my mother and dad's love and my dad's "never, ever give up" attitude that helped get me through it, survive, and rise again. I am eternally grateful for the lessons learned under their lifelong loving tutelage.

Erica Edell Phillips

Let me start with my wife and the love of my life, Erica. Erica and I have been together for more than three decades. Though we are not together as husband and wife just now, my love for her is as strong and real as the day I met her. Her steadfast commitment to my survival through the hardest of times and unceasing compassion during my illness and since, is the number one reason I am alive today. She took care of every single detail for me, medically and otherwise, and I don't think she had a full night's sleep during my treatment and many months thereafter, so busy was she worrying about me. Erica, I thank you every day for your help getting through those challenges—and many more—before and after. I am forever in your debt and will love you till the end of this lifetime and the next one and the next one.

Bridget Hough

Bridget, my "roomie" for the past three-plus years, is a remarkable woman with the courage to introduce herself and thank me for inspiring her with my keynote during her "Day One" orientation for new hires at UCLA Health. We became instant best friends. The rest, as they say, is history. Her amazing intelligence, exceptional kindness, generosity, beauty, hilarity, ethereal concert pianist skills, olive oil expertise, and endless compassion for me and countless others, buoys my spirits and helped heal my heart as I pursued my new life's purpose with the CARE Effect Movement. That and her great eyes and ears which resulted in her finding a five-week old abandoned tabby kitten we adopted and named Coco who has been an immense, shared joy for both of us.

Sarah Sheppeck
Then there is my brilliant cowriter on this project, Sarah "Shep" Sheppeck. Sarah is an exceptionally gifted writer and editor with the astonishing ability to take my written words and somehow not only improve them, but make them sound more like my actual voice than even I can. She is also perhaps the most patient human being on earth having put up with my perfectionism and endless rewrites to get this book done and into print. Thank you from the bottom of my heart, Shep, for both. I know you probably don't believe it, but we finally did it! Bless you for everything.

Shola Richards
Shola is my friend, my inspiration, fiercest friendly competitor, and role model. Before he left UCLA Health to become one of the world's best public

speakers and author of two of the best books on how to create kind, people-centric, and compassionate corporate cultures, Shola was responsible for the day-long orientations for all new hires at UCLA Health. Shola helped me start my post-cancer journey by inviting me to deliver weekly presentations on compassion to those UCLA Health new hires. Over four-plus years, I delivered more than two hundred for him and UCLA, and I am deeply thankful for that opportunity to hone my message and its delivery. After each week's presentation, we'd compare our audiences' written "reviews" to see who got the best ones. That friendly "competition" pushed me to continually improve, and I'm proud to say that eventually, I actually "won" a few times! You're the man.

Tony Padilla

Just after completing my cancer treatment and recovering sufficiently to again be able to speak, I had the great good fortune and privilege of being introduced to the hugely compassionate Anthony Padilla, then Tony, formerly the Chief of Patient Experience at UCLA Health, and now the Senior Vice President of Patient Experience at City of Hope Cancer Hospital. It was Tony who invited me onto UCLA Health's Patient Advisory Board and introduced me to Shola who then invited me to deliver weekly keynotes for over four years to every new UCLA hire during their Day One Orientation On-Boarding process. Tony's unending kindness, generosity of spirit, and support jump-started my speaking career at one of the most compassionate hospital systems in America (thanks in large part to his genius), which gave me the confidence and instant credibility to be able to reach out to other healthcare organizations and do the same. Thanks, Tony.

Barbara Christensen
Barbara's steadfast belief in me and my speaking skills, combined with a lot of hard work on my behalf through her Speak Well Being speaker bureau has brought dozens of prestigious speaking opportunities my way over the years. And, in doing so, helped turn my dream of helping improve the quality of care for patients and the healthcare providers who treat them into an ongoing enterprise. I can't thank you enough.

Daniel Ruark
Daniel is the "shrink" to the "stars" in Los Angeles, and though I certainly don't fit that category, he is in fact the "star" in my saga. It was Daniel with whom I had the privilege of speaking almost every single week for the past four to five years during the worst of the worst of all my miseries. The breakup with my wife Erica, my cancer treatment and its aftermath, the loss of my career, my fortune, my home, having to declare bankruptcy, and needing to drive for UBER to make ends meet. And, on the other side of the spectrum, the birth of the CARE Effect

Movement, my speaking work, cure, and personal reinvention into who I am and where I am happily today. Love you my friend and look forward to many rounds of golf and maybe a set or two of tennis *if* you take it easy on me.

Eli and Ari Gabayan, Lexi Timmons-Quintero, Andrew Budd, Narbeh Arkilian ...

... and all the other wonderful human beings at the Beverly Hills Cancer Center where I was gifted with the very best technical treatment *and* compassionate care when they beautifully treated, comforted, and cured me (woohoo!) and so many other deeply suffering cancer patients. Bless you all for who you are and what you do!

Art Snyder

Thank you my friend and brother from another mother for your support "every step" of the way during my recovery. You helped me reclaim my health and stamina inch-by-inch, step-by-step, and mile-by-mile on our post-treatment walks together. It wasn't easy, but you showing up day after day got me up, got me moving, and got me healthy again. Love you.

To Kim Thiboldeaux, Linda House and all your deeply kind and caring colleagues at the Cancer Support Community.

Your motto, "No one should go through cancer alone," is the epitome of compassion. Your combination of classes, support groups for patients and families, individual counseling, and sourcing information about everything to do with cancer, during and after, are nothing less than lifesaving and life-giving. And, *free!* I know because my wife and I used them all, and I continue to do so to this very day. Gilda Radner would be deeply proud of how you've taken her dream and expanded it nationwide. Bravo!